REPORT OF THE

CANCER SERVICES REVIEW

TO

THE LONDON IMPLEMENTATION GROUP

June 1993

London: HMSO

ISBN 0 11 321614 9

9308183

wx 150

CONTENTS

9. Significant Financial, Manpower and Implementation Issues

10. Appendices

1.1 TERMS OF REFERENCE

The Terms of Reference are set out in full in Appendix 1. Our principle task, as set out in Making London Better, has been 'to review specialist cancer services in London with the aim of achieving a more rational disposition, avoiding unwarranted duplication and providing a stronger service and academic base for the future'.

1.2 OUR APPROACH

Our approach has been that cancer services should be organised from the patient's perspective, with care, treatment and support being available through the primary, secondary and tertiary services on a coordinated basis. We have, therefore, made recommendations covering all these areas.

We have primarily considered the 11 specialist cancer units in central London. We have also, however, examined in some depth the four centres in outer London and the other six units in the South East, that is 21 centres in all, in order to clarify future referral patterns and so the likely size and stability of such centres.

1.3 THE CURRENT PICTURE

Incidence

We have assumed the current trend will continue and a 15% increase in the number of people with cancer will occur in next decade, due mainly to the increase in the number of elderly people and some small overall increases in incidence. For 1996/7 we have assumed there will be 62,000 new cancer cases within the 14.2M population of the four Thames Regions.

Referral patterns to specialist cancer centres in the South East

94% patients attending the 21 specialist centres in the South East live within the four Thames regions. The biggest inflow of patients (75%) is from the Oxford Region. We have assumed that 50% of this Region's inflow will disappear over the next five years. This will particularly affect the West London Units.

Referral patterns to London Units from within the Thames Regions

From the operation of the internal market and the new units already being created, a pattern already exists whereby more patients living in the South East, from outside London, are being treated at local units rather than travelling into London. We believe this trend will continue. This will also happen in the outskirts of London.

1.4 GENERAL CONCLUSIONS

<u>Undersized London Cancer Centres</u>

The 15 cancer centres in London only treat half the number of patients per annum of the average sized centre in the other 15 major metropolitan areas in the U.K. Taking a wider comparative sample of the 26 main centres in the rest of the UK, London units are still a third smaller on average.

<u>The variable quality of existing services</u>

From over 50 site visits and other analysis, it is clear that Londoners and others living in the South East are currently receiving a variable range and quality of cancer services. Not one single centre in the South East of England is at present offering everything that we believe can reasonably be expected from the NHS in the future, within present funding limits.

<u>Cancer specialists support the need for change</u>

The overwhelming majority of cancer specialists in London accept that the historic pattern of specialist centres needs major change and that a smaller number of larger centres would be more effective in delivering high quality service, teaching and research.

<u>Ending the current uncertainty</u>

Senior staff of the affected units and representatives of the local Health Authorities, RHAs, University and Cancer Research Organisations have all emphasised the need to avoid the current uncertainty being prolonged, with the risk of good staff leaving London.

<u>Safeguarding education and training</u>

Our proposals are designed to promote high quality undergraduate and postgraduate medical training in oncology and acknowledge the likely impact of the recent report of the CMO's Working Party on Specialist Training. London is also a major resource for training nurses at both basic and post basic levels, as well as radiographers and physicists and others who have important roles in cancer services. We have sought to identify actions to sustain these important activities.

-2-

<u>Support from the major cancer charities</u>

London has a prominent role in the national R & D programme for cancer which involves the major charities, MRC, and London University. Representatives from all these organisations have supported our general conclusion in favour of a smaller number of larger specialist centres in London, thereby giving them greater security for their investment in R & D.

1.5 DEFINING THE FUTURE SIZE AND NUMBER OF SPECIALIST CANCER CENTRES

<u>Accessibility</u>

The main objective of our proposals is that as much care as possible should be delivered locally, as long as it is of good quality. This underlies our proposals to strengthen the role of primary care and of services in local acute hospitals.

Our analysis of site options uses the criterion that 95% of patients should be able to reach a specialist cancer centre within one hour's travelling time.

<u>Problems of small Centres</u>

There are several serious disadvantages in the current pattern of small centres which the report sets out.

<u>Very large Centres</u>

Elsewhere in the country Specialist Centres exist that if recreated in London would mean the current 15 units might be reduced to as few as two or three, each treating up to 10,000 new (non-surgical) patients per year. The Review Group has concluded that there would be substantial disadvantages in this degree of centralisation, and we give reasons for this view.

<u>The proposed size of future London Centres</u>

The Review Group has concluded that the most appropriate model for Specialist Centres for London would be units seeing between 3,000 and 4,500 new clinical/medical oncology patients per annum.

The new centres we propose for London would be two to three times the average size of the present units but comparable in scale with those existing in most metropolitan centres elsewhere in the U.K.

<u>Appropriate staffing and equipment levels for London Centres</u>

Our Report sets out our proposals for the manpower and equipment required for high quality services to be provided by such centres within this size range, in the future.

<u>Specialist Centres outside central London</u>

The Review Group believes that it is desirable to retain and strengthen the existing pattern of cancer specialist centres outside the central London area. The proposals for the future pattern of such units is described in section 8 of the report.

<u>Inner London Centres</u>

The analysis of the options for the future patterns of specialist centres to replace the 11 that currently exist has been carried out on the basis that, apart from rare cancers that account for less than 10% of the total number of cases, people will be treated at their nearest Specialist Centre. London has been considered as being divided into four population sectors, or quadrants: North, North East, South East and the South West/West.

<u>Evaluation of options</u>

Given the number of existing units and the extent of recent capital investment, we do not see a case for any completely new cancer centres being built within the M25. We have, therefore, examined the relative suitability of existing sites using a number of factors described in the report, with the following conclusions.

1.6 THE NORTH EAST QUADRANT

St. Bartholomew's and the Royal London Hospitals are already working together as a 'shadow Trust' and have committed themselves to a single site specialist cancer centre. We endorse this objective.

The advantages of the Royal London site option are the anticipated retention of the widest range of specialties of any site in London, including a substantial volume of local acute services appropriate to the large population this hospital serves.

Whilst St. Bartholomew's Hospital's cancer services and research are of very high quality, we believe the site would be a poor choice for the North East London Cancer Centre given the advantages offered by the Royal London. The principal drawbacks of the St. Bartholomew's site are:-

-   The facilities for cancer services are so dispersed that even with a major capital investment a fully integrated unit could not be achieved.

-   A less complete range of regional specialties is available than at the Royal London.

-   The unit has a smaller local acute workload.

-   St. Bartholomew's has a much lower level of security within the health care market for the site overall.

We estimate the capital investment required at the Royal London site would be of the order of £11M and that it would take 2-3 years for a new North East London Centre to come into use. The unit would serve a population of some 1.1M people and treat some 3,600 new medical and clinical oncology patients per annum, with an associated broad base in surgical oncology.

1.7   THE SOUTH EAST QUADRANT

As long ago as 1982 the South East Thames RHA proposed that the three units of King's, Guy's and St. Thomas' should be merged into a single unit. This did not happen, but in 1985 unified management arrangements were introduced. Even so a partial range of cancer services has continued on all three sites and the fundamental drawbacks of the current arrangements are now even more clear than in the early 1980s. The Review Group has serious concerns about the provision of a radiotherapy service split over three sites and the detrimental effects this has in providing a patient focused service, for patient safety and for effective communications between patients and GPs.

These problems are understood by the consultants of all three hospitals, who support a move to a single site. The Review Group believes there is an urgent need to locate a specialist cancer service from these three hospitals on to one site. The Review has concluded that King's is the least suitable to become the future specialist cancer centre in the South East London because it is:-

-   The least accessible to the larger population to be served.

-   The smallest of the three.

-   It is not backed by such a substantial cancer sub-specialisation and research investment as the other two units.

-   King's management acknowledge that such an enlarged centre could only be provided by a completely new build. We do not believe that this is necessary given the quality of existing facilities at Guy's and St. Thomas'.

Although the balance of site selection between St. Thomas' and Guy's may well depend on other factors, the argument for cancer facilities alone we believe marginally favours the Guy's site, in spite of the radiotherapy department at St. Thomas' being the larger and the easier to expand. The particular points weighing in Guy's favour are:-

-   The strength of the current R & D and the investment made by other organisations in specialist facilities and staff.

-   The capacity for future R & D.

-   The highly effective integration of services and research for example in the breast cancer unit.

We estimate the capital investment required to locate all services on the Guy's site would be in the order of £10M and that it would take less than two years. The Unit would serve a population of approximately 1.25M and see some 4,000 new clinical/medical oncology patients per annum. This allows for the excellent, newly opened unit at Maidstone reversing some of the present patient flows into London.

1.8   THE SOUTH WESTERN/WESTERN QUADRANT

St. Mary's Hospital has the smallest radiotherapy and oncology service in London and acknowledges it will not remain a specialist cancer centre in the future. The other three larger centres, Charing Cross, the Hammersmith and the Royal Marsden (Fulham Road) are, all in the process of expanding their existing facilities. Yet this is the quadrant where it seems most likely that changes of referral patterns will reduce the demand for services in inner London and there is every prospect of significant spare capacity. In the short term, however, the combined workload of the three units would be above the maximum which we believe is appropriate for any one site and we propose that two centres should serve this part of London at present.

In recognition of the historic role fulfilled by the Royal Marsden Hospital and its high level of public support, our report examines in some detail the various issues which need to be resolved to give the best guarantee of this hospital having a secure and thriving future. Our conclusion is that the split site operation between the Sutton and Fulham Road branches (12 miles apart) has been a substantial drawback to the effective organisation of patient services, (mirroring some of the problems of the Guy's, King's and Thomas' quadrant). Also, travelling between the two sites severely limits the effectiveness of staff in their work and, we believe, their research and teaching potential.

Having examined various options, we recommend that the two branches of the Royal Marsden Hospital be consolidated on the Sutton site for the following reasons:-

-       The Sutton site already carries out almost two-thirds of the overall work of the unit and is the principal centre for treating most of the rare cancers referred to the Royal Marsden.

-       There is no other specialist cancer centre close to the Sutton Unit and it is, therefore, the most convenient referral centre for a large population in south west London and parts of Surrey. Its removal to the Fulham Road site would deprive this population of reasonable access to specialist cancer centres.

-       The Sutton site is ten times larger than that at Fulham Road and has a greater development potential, especially given that the Fulham Road site is already intensively developed.

To overcome the drawbacks of the Sutton unit not being a multi-specialty site, the Review recommends that a new Trust be formed combining St. George's Hospital and the Royal Marsden Hospital. We believe this is a preferable option to relying on the two separate Trusts achieving the necessary level of clinical and management integration. The new combined Trust would for example be better able to ensure the best balance between complex surgery being carried out on the St. George's and Sutton sites.

Should the unification of the Royal Marsden's services not proceed from Fulham to the Sutton site then the Review Group recommends that the Royal Marsden, Fulham Road be absorbed onto the Charing Cross Hospital site. This being the preferred location to the Hammersmith Hospital site, based on the following factors:-

-       Charing Cross has larger, more modern facilities.

-       It has good quality space available to accommodate those research units of the Royal Marsden Hospital that need to be close to clinical activities. (The basis of this need is addressed in our report).

-       Subject to the result of the other specialty reviews, Charing Cross will have a wider range of specialties than the Hammersmith site.

-       The Charing Cross staff have expressed a wish to become the major Specialist Centre serving west London, whereas staff at the Hammersmith expressed reservations about a large unit being appropriate, in terms of a balanced wide range of moderately sized specialties, to support its overall research and postgraduate teaching role.

- The site constraints at the Hammersmith are substantially greater than those on the Charing Cross site and would, therefore, involve higher cost and might result in a less satisfactory pattern of facilities than the Charing Cross site.

For similar reasons the Review Group has concluded that Charing Cross would be the preferred site for the major cancer centre for west London. It is assumed that the unit will increase in size by some 500 cases from the current level of 3,000 new clinical/medical oncology cases per annum as a consequence of our recommendation that the Royal Marsden consolidates its services at Sutton, and some of its Chelsea patients will, therefore, more naturally go to Charing Cross. This estimate also takes into account some reduction of referrals into West London from East Berkshire, and that some of the catchment of the old Westminster cancer centre, e.g. the Maidstone area, will not follow its recent relocation to Charing Cross.

We recommend that the Hammersmith Hospital service be retained and that the new high quality facilities be better utilised by building on existing links with St. Mary's.

Given the wide range of uncertainties surrounding this part of London, we suggest that a further review is carried out within three years to reassess the most appropriate future pattern of services, having regard to the referral patterns then apparent.

1.9 THE NORTH LONDON QUADRANT

The services currently provided by UCH/Middlesex and the Royal Free hospitals are more satisfactory than in some other quadrants and there are no site closure issues which demand that urgent action is taken.

The UCH/Middlesex service is about three times the size of that of the Royal Free.

There are already effective working links, in particular between the medical oncology units of the two hospitals and we recommend that these are further promoted by the two medical schools also coming closer together, as we believe is planned.

The two hospitals also both have large haematology services and it is likely that in the future only one highly specialised unit will be required, not least in terms of cost, in this part of London.

The recommendation of the Review Group is that plans should be developed, subject to a further detailed appraisal, to base the North

London Specialist Cancer Centre at the Middlesex Hospital serving a population of 1.15M with some 3,600 new clinical/medical oncology patients being treated per annum. The capital costs would be of the order of £3M. Should it be proposed that for reasons related to the capacity of the Middlesex Unit or on other grounds a new unit be developed on the UCH site, the Review Group would expect the option of maintaining and expanding services of the Royal Free to be also thoroughly examined.

The Review Group recognises the attractions of the Royal Free site in terms that it is more modern and open than the UCH/Middlesex campus, generally having more flexibility for development and a sounder record of financial management. However, the Review Group has placed greater weight on issues directly concerned with cancer services.

The principal reasons for favouring the centralisation at the Middlesex rather than at the Royal Free site are:-

-       As it is three times the size, moderate expansion to the projected size will be easier than the larger expansion that would be necessary on the Royal Free site.

-       That the range and the quality of research activities associated with the UCH/Middlesex unit are more substantial than those of the Royal Free.

-       That the presence of a major cancer centre on the UCH/Middlesex site will attract further high calibre research, funding given the proximity of University College.

1.10 UNITS IN OUTER LONDON AND OTHER PARTS OF SOUTH EAST ENGLAND

We have concluded, after on-site discussions with local staff, that the units at Southend, Canterbury and Brighton will remain serving populations that do not look to London for specialist cancer services to any significant extent.

We anticipate that the excellent new Maidstone unit opened in April at a cost of £23M will attract a substantial number of patients who have, up to now, been referred to centres in London. Similarly, the large centre that already exists at Guildford and which is now being redeveloped on the Royal Surrey site at a cost of £12M will have a similar, but less marked, impact on London units.

Both the Colchester and Oldchurch Units in the North East Thames Region are small centres that require redevelopment. We believe serious consideration should be given to a single, better staffed and equipped, larger centre being built at an appropriate geographical location, perhaps

Chelmsford, rather than that each of these small units should be separately replaced. Such a new unit would marginally increase referrals into North and East London (the London Hospital and the North Middlesex).

The Review has concluded that the three other Centres in outer London should all be retained as described below.

The Unit at the North Middlesex has an appreciable catchment area north of London and should be expanded to a modest extent to serve a population of about 900,000 people and treat some 2,500 new clinical/ medical oncology patients per annum.

The Mount Vernon unit being the largest in the South East of England should remain at much its current size.

The services spread across the two branches of the Royal Marsden Hospital in Fulham Road and Sutton should be consolidated on the latter site, which would, therefore, require some development as described earlier in this summary in order to provide a comprehensive service to its local south west London and Surrey population, whilst maintaining its special clinical expertise and its research base. It should establish firm formal links with St. George's, as previously described.

Paediatric oncology is addressed by the Children's specialty review. We believe that children's needs for radiotherapy, as proposed by that review, are fully compatible with our own recommendations.

An appraisal of capital and revenue consequences of these proposals is included in the Report. Some revenue savings will be achieved. The extra capital needed will not be greatly more than would be required for maintaining the current number of smaller centres, and should be amply met by site sales. The benefits of the new arrangements to patients will be considerable.

Sector	Current Sites	Recommended Sites	Timescale	Other Options Considered
North East Quadrant	The Royal London St. Bartholomew's	Establish the North East London centre, at The Royal London to serve a population of 1.1M	As the unit will be substantially a new build, not estimated to be open until 1996/7. Estimated cost is £11M	1. Centralise at St. Bartholomew's and close The Royal London unit. 2. Status quo
	Colchester, Oldchurch and Southend units	Create a new Essex unit to avoid undersized redevelopments at Oldchurch and Colchester. Southend to continue.	Estimated cost £16M. RHA to organise review of site options to be completed by December 1993. Open by 1996/97.	1. Close Southend as well and create a single Essex unit, i.e. 3 into 1 2. Redevelop separately the existing Colchester and Oldchurch units.
South East Quadrant	Guy's, King's and St. Thomas's	Guy's to become South East London centre serving 1.25M	Open within two years after radiotherapy department expansion has been achieved at circa £10M King's could close by April 1994. The disruption of Guy's services during redevelopment might justify retention until 1995/96 of the King's unit.	1. Centralise on King's site. 2. Centralise on St. Thomas's site.

Sector	Current Sites	Recommended Sites	Timescale	Other Options Considered
South Western/ Western Quadrant	Royal Marsden, the Hammersmith, Charing Cross and St. Mary's	Charing Cross to be the main unit for West London. The new unit would serve one million people and be linked to the Hammersmith unit which will expand to serve approximately 750,000 people. The Royal Marsden, Sutton Branch to be expanded and absorb some of the Fulham Road work. New joint Trust to be formed of the Royal Marsden and St. George's.	Relocation of Fulham Road Branch to the Sutton likely to cost £6M mainly for additional R & D facilities. Could be achieved within two years. Expenditure required at Charing Cross and Hammersmith for modest expansion not likely to be more than £2M in total.	1. Marsden to continue on two sites. 2. Centralise all Marsden work at Fulham Road. 3. Absorb Marsden work at Hammersmith compared with Charing Cross option.
	Mount Vernon	To remain much the same size	RHA organised review of possible northern unit and local acute services pattern to be completed by December 1993.	

Sector	Current Sites	Recommended Sites	Timescale	Other Options Considered
Northern Quadrant	The Royal Free UCH/Middlesex	Create an enlarged unit on the Middlesex site. Cost £3M. If North Middlesex not to be expanded, re-examine advantages of a possible UCH rebuild against an extension of the Royal Free facilities.	Less urgent than some quadrants. Clarify options by April 1994. Implement single site options over next two to four years.	1. Centralise at the Royal Free. 2. Status quo. 3. Close North Middlesex unit.
	North Middlesex	Expand to serve population of 800,000 at cost up to £1.5M.	Within one year	

LOCATION OF 15 SPECIALIST CANCER CENTRES IN LONDON

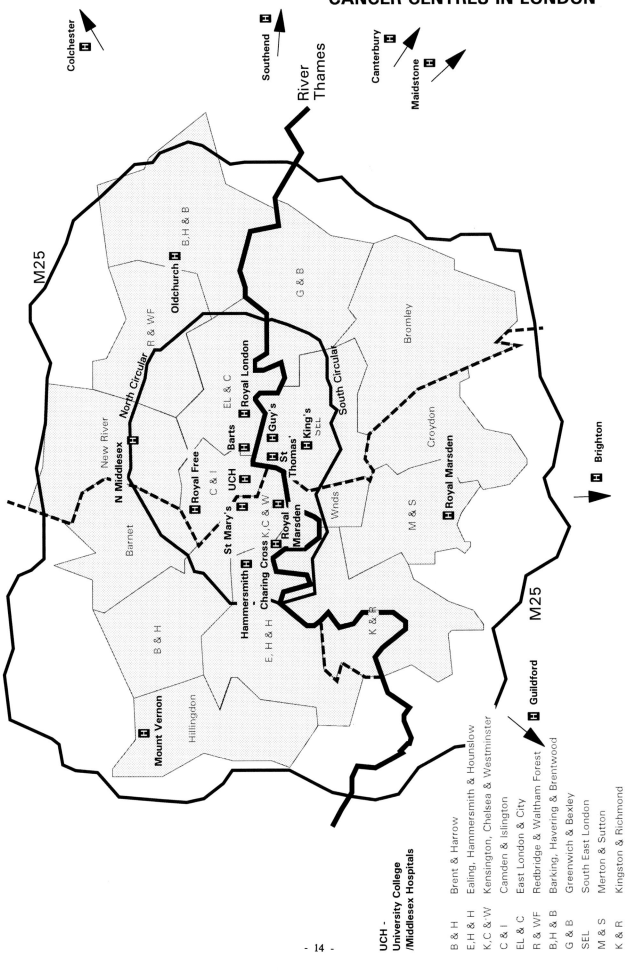

UCH -
University College
/Middlesex Hospitals

B & H   Brent & Harrow
E,H & H   Ealing, Hammersmith & Hounslow
K,C & W   Kensington, Chelsea & Westminster
C & I   Camden & Islington
EL & C   East London & City
R & WF   Redbridge & Waltham Forest
B,H & B   Barking, Havering & Brentwood
G & B   Greenwich & Bexley
SEL   South East London
M & S   Merton & Sutton
K & R   Kingston & Richmond

- 14 -

SUMMARY OF RECOMMENDATIONS

General recommendations - the interface between primary care and specialist centres

That a small working party comprising representatives of patients, voluntary patient support organisations, the professions, Community Health Councils, provider units and local Health Authorities should be set up to develop a National Charter for cancer patients, within a six month period. **(page 33)**

That Health Authorities and service providers should take active measures to ensure equitable access to services for all sections of the local population. **(page 34)**

That action should be taken to improve the accuracy of FHSA registration data and target groups with a low uptake of breast and cervical screening. **(page 35)**

That the Royal College of General Practitioners in conjunction with the Royal College of Nursing should take a lead in ensuring that continuing education programmes for GPs and nurses include the diagnosis of cancer. **(page 36)**

That the initiative of the Royal Colleges of Physicians and Radiologists in proposing targets for rapid access to hospital diagnostic and treatment services for cancer patients should be supported and extended. **(page 36)**

That DHAs/FHSAs should set minimum standards for the content and speed of communications from hospitals to GPs and Community Nursing Teams, and monitor the quality of information provided. **(page 36)**

That Health Authorities should review their palliative care services with a view to improving them, particularly for patients who wish to remain at home. **(page 38)**

That Specialist Cancer Centres should have a leadership role in improving cancer services overall, working in conjunction with other providers within the NHS and those in the voluntary sector. **(page 39)**

That local Health Authorities should work with the Specialist Cancer Centres to ensure better co-ordinated local services are introduced, as quickly as possible, and be subject to systematic clinical, managerial and consumer audits. **(page 39)**

That innovative schemes to help patients deal with travelling problems should be adopted more generally. **(page 47)**

Improving care at Specialist Centre level

That Cancer Centres should be created that are of a size to treat some 3,000 - 4,500 new non-surgical oncology patients per year; this size best supporting both patient care and research and development. **(page 48)**

That cancer centres should be on the same site as, and have the advantages of the multiple available services and skills of major general hospitals. **(pages 51, 52)**

That clinical cancer research is also best located with general hospital research activity. **(page 52)**

That basic science cancer research is usually best linked most strongly to University science departments, not necessarily on hospitals sites. **(page 41)**

That for an average-sized local acute hospital, consultant cancer specialists should be available on site for most days of the working week and on call for urgent consultation. **(page 39)**

That greater surgical specialisation should be applied to the care of many cancers, common and less common. **(page 40)**

That major surgery for gynaecological cancers should be carried out by a greater degree of specialisation. **(page 40)**

That a task group should be set up to develop detailed proposals on improving information systems on cancer services by April 1994 with implementation, after some market testing, no later than April 1995. **(page 44)**

That bed numbers should be reviewed periodically in the light of the trend towards more day care as against the growing number of elderly people with multi-system disease needing inpatient care. **(page 50)**

That, given the number of existing units and the extent of recent capital investment, there is no case for any completely new Cancer Centres being built within the M25. **(page 60)**

That the four Thames Regions consider extending joint commissioning arrangements for radiography training. **(page 126)**

That haematology services for the treatment of blood related malignancies should be reviewed with a view to achieving a smaller number of larger specialist units, when the decisions arising from the present review are known. **(page 105)**

SECTOR ANALYSIS

North East London Quadrant

That the adult cancer services at St. Bartholomew's hospital should be moved to and combined with those at the Royal London hospital. **(page 64)**

That a commitment to a substantial capital scheme, on the Royal London site, of the order of £11M needs to be given, as a matter of priority, if the service to people in the North Eastern Quadrant of London is to match the physical facilities already available in some other quadrants of London. An early decision should be made on this investment to prevent the groups of high quality staff based at St. Bartholomew's Hospital from breaking up. **(page 65)**

South East London Quadrant

That the two Radiotherapy Units at St Thomas' and Guy's Hospitals should be consolidated onto one site, and the King's Radiotherapy Unit should close. **(pages 71,72)**

South Western/Western London Quadrant

That the two branches of the Royal Marsden Hospital be consolidated on the Sutton site. **(page 96)**

That a new Trust be formed combining the Royal Marsden Hospital and St. George's Hospital, and a carefully planned process of change set in motion. **(pages 94,96)**

That should the unification of the Royal Marsden's services not proceed from Fulham to the Sutton site, then the Royal Marsden Fulham Road be absorbed onto the Charing Cross Hospital site. This is regarded as a less desirable option than unifying the Royal Marsden on its main (Sutton) site. **(pages 93,117,118)**

That the Hammersmith Hospital site be retained as a cancer centre and that the new high quality facilities be better utilised by building on existing links with St. Mary's. **(page 95)**

That a review be undertaken of the current pattern of split surgical appointments at the Hammersmith Hospital with a view to increasing the level of on-site surgical commitment and sub-specialisation. **(page 80)**

That, as currently proposed, the Chelsea Health Sciences Centre would not resolve the underlying problems facing the Royal Marsden Hospital. But that there would be great advantage in a wider group of Institutions within West

London (including Hammersmith and Charing Cross) forming a closer relationship with Imperial College, as well as the Institute of Cancer Research. **(page 87)**

That research links be strengthened between the Charing Cross Unit, RPMS/Hammersmith, Imperial College and the Institute of Cancer Research. **(pages 79,81)**

That the Hammersmith Hospital's cancer services develop closer working links with the expanded Charing Cross Unit. **(page 90)**

That the North West Thames RHA and Local Health Authorities, in conjunction with national research and teaching interests, should review within three years the roles being fulfilled by the two remaining Cancer Centres in West London, namely the Hammersmith and Charing Cross Units. **(page 96)**

The North London Quadrant

That plans should be developed, subject to a further detailed appraisal, to base the North London Specialist Cancer Centre at the Middlesex Hospital with the Radiotherapy Unit at the Royal Free Hospital closing. **(page 102)**

That the Royal Free should continue to have a large Haematology Unit but without on-site radiotherapy. The development of high dose chemotherapy for solid tumours may be best concentrated on the Middlesex site. **(page 103)**

Outer London

Southend, Canterbury and Brighton Units to continue to serve the populations that are remote from London. **(pages 107,108,112)**

That a new Essex Radiotherapy Unit be considered to avoid reproviding two small units at Colchester and Oldchurch, both of which now require closure and relocation to general hospital sites. **(page 111)**

That the Unit at the North Middlesex Hospital be expanded to a modest extent. **(page 114)**

That the North East Thames RHA, with the relevant local Health Authorities, should immediately set up a review to identify whether the rebuilding of two small Centres at Colchester and Oldchurch, can be justified in capital investment terms, and more importantly service quality terms, as opposed to a single, more comprehensive Centre being built. **(pages 112,113)**

That the Unit at Mount Vernon Hospital should remain at much its current size subject to a review. **(page 120)**

That the combined CT/Simulator installed at Mount Vernon be the subject of a Health Technology Assessment exercise by the Department of Health. **(page 119)**

More distant centres

That the South East Thames RHA and local Health Authorities review the DGHs to which Maidstone Unit could be linked by June 1994. **(page 106)**

That a longterm site development plan for the Brighton Unit be worked out. **(page 108)**

That a review be undertaken by North West Thames, Oxford and East Anglia RHAs as to how best cancer patients in the areas of Bedford, Milton Keynes, Luton, Stevenage and Hitchin should be served. The evaluation of options should be completed no later than December 1993. **(page 111)**

That links between the Colchester and Southend Units should be strengthened. **(page 113)**

2.1   INCIDENCE

Cancer is common: we are all at risk. National statistics show that one in three people will develop cancer at some time in their lives, and that one in four will die from it.

It is becoming more common, mainly because it occurs more frequently with advancing age, and our population is ageing.

Lung, skin, breast and gastrointestinal cancer account for half of the cases and with others form a diverse range of some 200 different cancer types. Nevertheless a concentration of skills common to all is needed in prevention, early diagnosis, treatment and palliative care.

2.2   PREVENTION, CARE AND TREATMENT

The importance of the targets set in "Health of the Nation" for preventing cancer, and for improving cure rate through earlier diagnosis and treatment, cannot be stressed sufficiently. Our Review Group supports them most strongly. The main thrust of this Review is however to underpin these targets by improving the care of patients with cancer in London, now, and into the next century.

2.3   RELATIVELY MODEST SURVIVAL IMPROVEMENTS

Our proposals are made in the context that although survival rates for several forms of cancer have much improved over the past 20 years, the overall advances have been relatively modest. The really major improvements have mainly been in treating rarer cancers that account for less than 10% of the total. Nevertheless, further improvements can be made using existing therapies, providing that services are better organised. Palliative and terminal care have improved greatly over this period. They are directed to improving the quality of life of patients who must live with their cancer, and to relieving symptoms.

2.4   NEW TREATMENTS

The advice of cancer specialists working within and outside London, also of other Clinical Directors of Cancer Centres in the U.K., and from leaders in current cancer research, is that it is unlikely that there will be a single breakthrough in the next 5-10 years which will make a dramatic impact in improving survival rates, let alone a set of new treatments which will replace those now available (surgery, radiotherapy and chemotherapy), across the whole diverse range of cancers that exist. We recognise the major input which will be made in the longer term by emerging technologies. These include improved and more accurate diagnosis through advances in imaging (MRI) and immunodiagnostics, and new potential gene therapies and molecular medicine through advancing our knowledge of cell biology. Other technical improvements in existing treatments will continue and will also prove valuable. But the usefulness of these advances will, on wide advice we have had, take some years to be realised in practice. (Wilkie, T. 'Perilous Knowledge' 1993)

2.5 INCREASING INCIDENCE

The assumption made in this report is there will be a 15% increase in the number of people with cancer over the next decade, mainly due to the increased number of elderly people, (70% of people with cancer are aged over 60), but also due to small overall increases in incidence. This assumption includes an allowance for an increased demand for treatment from patients not currently receiving it, as education and awareness develop, and earlier diagnosis is achieved.

2.6 U.K. SURVIVAL RATES

An analysis by the World Health Organisation (1988) showed that the female population of the U.K., aged under 65, ranked the second highest in cancer death rate of the 16 industrial countries surveyed - mainly due to high rates of breast and lung cancer. The male U.K. population under 65 ranked 7th out of 16. These and other differences in survival rates between the U.K. and other countries have been given much publicity. These are however certainly due in part to epidemiological differences and selection bias. The role of the quality of treatment is very difficult to establish, and in our belief there is insufficient evidence to support the claim that cancer services in the U.K. are poorer, or conversely better, than in comparable countries.

2.7 OUTCOME: CURE AND QUALITY OF LIFE

It would be widely agreed that the provision of cancer services should be related to their outcome for the patient and family. In theory this is easy to measure by such indices as survival rate. In practice however such crude measures are not very helpful in a condition where quality of life during treatment and for those who are not cured, are so very important.

We believe that the current interest in improving the scientific basis of measures of quality of care should be strongly supported. It should perhaps include the measurement of patients' view by means such as the American SF36 scoring system. We do not however think that the outcome measures that currently exist are sufficiently developed or sensitive to be of general applicability in determining policies for cancer care.

2.8   CANCER DATA

We are very aware that the data available to us whether in terms of cancer statistics, outcomes, activity or costs, available to us has been imperfect. We regard the correction of this problem, which has faced all previous cancer service reviews in London or elsewhere, as a major challenge for the future. With contracting, this will be ever more important.

3.1 A COORDINATED PLAN

Our approach has been that cancer services should be organised from the patient's perspective, with care, treatment and support being available through the primary, secondary and tertiary services, on a co-ordinated basis. We do not believe that decisions for change can properly be based on a study of the Specialist Cancer Centres on their own, and so have made recommendations across all these areas.

3.2 SPECIALIST CENTRES IN INNER LONDON

We have principally considered the specialist hospital services for cancer patients in the 11 units in central London. However referral patterns are so slanted by history, and the likely impact of good quality, often new Cancer Centres elsewhere in the South East is so marked, that we have considered in some depth the four units in outer London, as well as briefly examining six other units in the South East, i.e. 21 units in all. (The role of the Reading and Northampton Units and two private units, at the Cromwell and Midhurst, has also been considered).

Inner London Centres (11)	Outer London Units, but still inside the M25 (4)	Other Units in the South East (6)
St. Bartholomew's The Royal London King's, Guy's & St.Thomas's The Royal Marsden (Fulham) Hammersmith Charing Cross St. Mary's UCH/Middlesex Royal Free	North Middlesex Oldchurch The Royal Marsden (Sutton) Mount Vernon	Colchester Southend Canterbury Maidstone Brighton Guildford

3.3 PREVIOUS REPORTS

There have been over a dozen reports on cancer services since 1970, most central (DoH) guidance dates from that decade. In the 1980s the Thames Region commissioned a number of reviews and in the late 1980s and early 1990s more comprehensive reviews have been undertaken of

Scottish and Welsh services, as well as by some English Regions, e.g. the South Western and Northern RHAs (see bibliography).

Most of the reports have confirmed that the organisation of cancer services should follow the following broad principles:-

-   Comprehensive Cancer Centres of excellence should have good links and communication with local hospital services.

-   Radiotherapy and Medical Oncology should be integrated within Cancer Centres which should deliver a full service to cancer patients.

-   Cancer Units in local acute Hospitals should be well linked with Cancer Centres, cancer registration and research organisation.

-   Sound monitoring mechanisms and information systems for audit and evaluation should exist.

-   Cancer Centres should provide a regular, organised consultancy service for local acute hospitals and co-ordinate teaching and research.

4.1   CONFIRMATION OF THE TOMLINSON ANALYSIS

Sir Bernard Tomlinson's conclusions about London's health service are confirmed by this Review for cancer services, namely:-

-        That a higher level of resources is being spent in London than the rest of the country, exemplified by there being:-

    -        more specialist cancer beds;
    -        more equipment;
    -        more medical and paramedical staff.

The scale of greater provision ranges from 10% for consultant staff, to well over 50% for major treatment equipment.

-        Co-ordination between primary, secondary and tertiary care is under-developed.

4.2   UNDERSIZED LONDON CANCER CENTRES

The Cancer Centres in London are on average under half the size of Specialist Units in other large Metropolitan areas in the U.K. (This is taking the 15 largest cities in the U.K. that have Cancer Centres as the comparative group). The average London unit treated 1800 new radiotherapy and non surgical oncology patients per year, whilst the average for the Centres in other main Metropolitan areas has 3700 (1990 figures).

Taking a wider sample of 26 Centres serving urban areas, the Specialist Cancer Units in London still treated on average a third less patients: 1800 new cases per annum, compared with 2,800 for the rest of the U.K. These comparisons are based on data provided from a survey carried out in 1990 by the Royal College of Radiologists.

We have obtained 1992 data from a sample of Centres outside London, which has allowed a comparison to be made with the more recent figures of the London Centres. This confirms that the difference in size has persisted, and even widened slightly.

4.3   VARIATIONS IN RESOURCE USE

The differences in the effective use of staff, equipment and other resources are marked between London units as the table below shows.

REVIEW OF LONDON'S CANCER SERVICES	RANGE OF WORKLOAD PER ANNUM			
SUMMARY RATIOS OF CURRENT ACTIVITY	HIGHEST	MEAN	LOWEST	MEDIAN
STAFFING RATIOS				
New oncology patterns per WTE oncology consultant	661	380	236	456
Radiotherapy courses per WTE therapy radiographer	173	115	78	118
WTE radiographers per radiotherapy machine	3.44	2.31	1.25	2.48
Radiotherapy courses per WTE physicist	919	439	203	447
WTE physicists per radiotherapy machine	0.89	0.60	0.43	0.67
RADIOTHERAPY EQUIPMENT				
Radiotherapy courses per new oncology patient	1.31	1.08	0.66	1.17
Courses per megavoltage machine per annum	864	573	254	610
Courses per simulator per annum	3,715	2,049	1,016	2,102
BEDS				
New clinical oncology cases per available bed	124	40	24	60
Average length of inpatient stay - days	10.5	7.1	3.6	8.7
Inpatient bed days per new oncology patient	11.3	6.7	2.6	8.0
CHEMOTHERAPY				
Doses per patient	25	12	2	6
Doses per pharmacist	4,640	2,039	630	1,810

Commentary on Table

These wide variations surprised the Review Group. Some have explanations that seem reasonable in terms of special services or research, but the overall range is greater than can be accounted for by these factors.

A further illustration of this diversity, only partly attributed in our view to wide variations in costing methodology, are the ECR tariffs for cancer services shown in the following table:-

ECR TARIFFS FOR CANCER SERVICES (£)

	Radiotherapy		Medical Oncology	
	In-patient episode	Day Care	In-patient episode	Day Care
Charing Cross	*	*	3235	338
UCH/Middlesex	4073	445	2352	530
Guy's/Thomas'	N/K	N/K	584	262
Royal Free	1869	218	1994	214
St.Bart's	874-3507	*	1161-4692	353
Royal London	1171	165	Up to 5699	*
Mt.Vernon	*	140	*	275
Nth. Middx.	1633	921	1633	921

*   Not comparable since charges not calculated by episode.

4.4 CAPITAL INVESTMENT

The current pattern of a large number of small specialist Cancer Centres in the South East of England has led to capital investment being thinly spread. Few Centres have a comprehensive set of modern buildings and equipment, or the necessary range of specialist staff for the future. (A sum in excess of £80M has nevertheless been spent in the last five years; the investment being in the order of £3M/£4M per site. The two Royal Marsden sites have had some £45M spent on capital schemes.) Many sites still have poor quality facilities e.g. utilitarian outpatient areas, wards offering low levels of privacy, some old equipment, and frequently cytotoxic drug preparation areas that are inadequate. Others on the other hand have facilities that are first rate.

The Review Group has concluded that the facilities suitable for treating cancer in the 21st century can only be achieved by investment, in people as well as physical facilities, being concentrated on a substantially smaller number of sites. The Review Group believes that in future a higher proportion of the money spent on cancer services should be invested in staff, with expenditure on capital being concentrated to provide the very best quality facilities, used more cost-effectively than now.

4.5 CURRENT SERVICES ARE OF VARIABLE QUALITY

The Review has involved over 50 site visits (at least 3 to each London Centre), and numerous individual discussions with cancer specialists and research workers, as well as detailed work by six separate study groups. Our overall conclusion is that Londoners, and others living in the South East, are currently receiving a more variable range and quality of cancer services than they should, or need to do. Many examples of good practice and excellence have been identified, and the Review has drawn these together into a model of service that we believe will offer higher quality, better co-ordinated care, than is currently available. Most of what we have recommended already exists somewhere in the South East, but no one centre is at present offering everything we believe can reasonably be expected from the NHS in the future, within present funding limits.

4.6 CANCER SPECIALISTS SUPPORT THE NEED FOR MAJOR CHANGE

The overwhelming majority of cancer specialists have confirmed that the historic pattern needs major change with fewer Centres in future, to create better services for patients, and to provide an improved basis for teaching and clinical research to achieve high standards.

4.7 MANAGING THE CHANGES

Senior staff of the London units we have visited, local Health Authority representatives, RHAs, University representatives and the Cancer Research Organisations, have all emphasised the need to implement the required changes without delay, thereby avoiding prolonged drift and uncertainty, and the risk of good staff leaving London. Our proposals will involve substantial change for many staff, and the Review Group believes that this will require sophisticated management.

We are very aware of the complex mix of skills and facilities that characterises many of the excellent specialist services now offered. These must not be allowed to disintegrate by either lack of decision, or insufficiently careful planning for change.

4.8 SAFEGUARDING EDUCATION AND TRAINING

The major role of the London Cancer Centres in the Nation's training plans will also need care in reorganisation. These Centres currently have 56 recognised training posts in clinical oncology, 20 in medical oncology, many in surgery where sub-specialisation in oncology is a strong feature, and in haematology. The proposals in this report are designed to foster high quality postgraduate training, and acknowledge the impact of the recent report of the CMO's Working Party on Specialist Training. The diagnosis and management of cancer patients should be an integral element in undergraduate medical training. It is important that arrangements are made to ensure that all medical schools have close links with tertiary cancer centres.

London also provides a major resource for training nurses (both basic and post basic courses), radiographers, physicists, physiotherapists, and others who support cancer services. Patterns of care and skill-mix are likely to change greatly in future. Training will be of the utmost importance for an effective response to be made to these changes.

4.9 SUPPORT FROM THE MAJOR RESEARCH ORGANISATIONS

The particular role of London in the national R & D programme for cancer, involving NHS R & D, the major and many smaller charities, the M.R.C., and London University, will be a complex area requiring different Central Government departments to co-operate in implementing these changes.

The representatives of the larger research organisations to whom we have spoken have supported our general conclusions in favour of a smaller number of larger specialist Centres in London, giving greater security for their investment in research and development.

4.10 THE NEED FOR MAJOR CAPITAL INVESTMENT

Net additional capital investment (approximately £30M) will be needed over a 5 year period if the current relatively inefficient, unnecessarily expensive service, is to be replaced by the somewhat more centralised and significantly more effective pattern we propose. But simply to maintain the current diffuse pattern would, we calculate, be at least as expensive if acceptable levels of safety and service are to be provided. Taking both these factors into account, we believe that the re-arrangements we propose would cost no more than necessary capital replacements that would be needed to continue the existing large number of small Centres, over a ten year period. Furthermore, fewer sites will realise estates savings and, in our view, bring improved patient care and research potential.

4.11 THE LACK OF AN EFFECTIVE INFORMATION SYSTEM

The most difficult problem encountered by the Review Team has been the lack of comparable data for all aspects of cancer services. This is considered in section 5.4 and in Appendix 4, where we make recommendations for improvements that we consider to be of the utmost importance for the future.

4.12 THE ROLE OF VOLUNTARY AND RESEARCH ORGANISATIONS IN CANCER SERVICES

The role fulfilled by the Voluntary and Charitable organisations in support of the cancer services of the NHS has been, and continues to be, invaluable. It will need to be considered carefully so that it may be built upon as the NHS changes we are proposing are put into effect.

The extent to which cancer services for people in the South East of England are provided by the NHS in partnership with these other organisations is well illustrated by the following:

-      Some 21% of consultant clinical and medical oncology posts are funded by non-NHS sources (principally University posts and those of the MRC and major cancer charities). Within this overall figure 12% of consultant radiotherapy posts and 40% of consultant medical oncology posts in London are funded from non-NHS sources.

-      Some 80% of hospice beds are provided by a network of voluntary organisations, many of which are local groups.

-      Two-thirds of the home care and three-quarters of day care cancer services across the Thames Regions are provided by voluntary organisations.

-      Cancer research is substantially funded by the major cancer research charities: the Imperial Cancer Research Fund, the Cancer Research Campaign and the Leukaemia Research Fund. Much support is also provided by local Council Research Funds and by industry, especially pharmaceutical companies and equipment manufacturers.

-      The Department of Health funds some research directly, and central Government also provides considerable support via the UFC (to London University), and through the Medical Research Council.

This pluralistic pattern of funding and delivering services has been a longstanding feature of cancer services, rather than a recent trend. The Imperial Cancer Research Fund was founded in 1902, the Macmillan Foundation in 1911, the Cancer Research Campaign in 1923 and the Marie Curie Foundation became operational, like the NHS, in 1948.

As indicated in 'Making London Better' (paragraph 37) there is a need to develop the Voluntary Sector further. This is especially important for cancer services, where the current arrangements are very variable across London.

A brief description of the distinctive roles of some of these voluntary and charitable organisations, which have achieved so much for cancer patients, follows. It is hoped that this may help some of those who work in the NHS to understand them better and thereby be able to plan and deliver services more effectively in conjunction with their support.

The Cancer Relief Macmillan Fund (CRMF)

- Priority is support to patients and families.
- Funds specialist nursing posts and lectureships.
- Pump-primes service developments in conjunction with local Health Authority.
- Gives grants to patients in financial need.
- Provides capital to launch day care and in-patient facilities. This capital is returned to Cancer Relief by local fundraising.
- Jointly funds Regional Nursing Co-ordination posts.
- Funds medical posts at Consultant, Senior Registrar, Registrar and SHO levels.
- Funds education programmes for nurses and doctors in areas such as pain control.
- Funds GP facilitation schemes to increase GP's knowledge and understanding of palliative care.

The Imperial Cancer Research Fund (ICRF)

- Funds a third of cancer research in the U.K.
- Annual support for research amounts to some £50M.
- 64% of research funding goes into laboratories for molecular biology and other aspects of cancer research.
- 36% of research funding goes into hospital-based research and cancer prevention.
- Funds laboratory and clinically based cancer research.
- Central laboratories in Lincoln's Inn Fields.
- Other established research units at the interface between the laboratory and clinics at several major Cancer Centres in the country.
- Supports large units at St. Bartholomew's and the Hammersmith Hospital, and smaller units at some other London Centres.
- Its continued support is dependent upon regular external review of research outcome and effectiveness.

The Cancer Research Campaign (CRC)

- Funds a third of cancer research in the U.K.
- Annual support for research amounts to some £47M; 36% of which (£17M) goes to London based research.
- Funds both laboratory and clinically based research.
- 42% of total research funding goes to four Research Institutions - the Beatson Institute (Glasgow), the Institute for Cancer Research (The Royal Marsden), the Paterson Institute (Manchester) and the CRC Gray Laboratory (Mount Vernon).
- 49% of research funding linked to universities and medical schools. Substantial grants to University College and UCH/Middlesex School of Medicine, Charing Cross and Westminster Medical School, St. George's Hospital Medical School, the Royal Free Hospital School of Medicine, the Royal Postgraduate Medical School, King's College School of Medicine and Dentistry, and a number of other medical schools and colleges in London.
- 5% of funding is in the form of personal awards; fellowships, studentships and grants.
- £1.5M allocated to psychological and educational research.
- Continued support is dependent upon regular external review of research outcome and effectiveness.

Marie Curie Memorial Foundation (MCMF)

- Runs eleven Centres in the U.K. (two in the Thames Regions), providing day care and in-patient services, and also in service training and some clinical placements for other professionals.
- Funds the Marie Curie Research Institute, Oxted, Surrey, specialising in molecular genetics.
- Funds the Marie Curie Education Department which organises courses, conferences, seminars and workshops all over the U.K. for health care professionals and others working in Cancer Care.
- Together with local Health Authorities, funds nurses of all grades to work with community nurses providing home nursing to people with cancer and support to carers.

THREE PARALLEL APPROACHES

The conclusion of the Review Group is that an improved quality of life and survival rates from cancer requires three parallel approaches:-

A better balanced and co-ordinated service - In the short term it has to be accepted that working within the current limits of medical knowledge, the major objective is to provide a better organised, higher quality service. One third of cancer patients can only be appropriately offered palliative care, and so cancer services are as much about improving the quality of life as prolonging it.

A better organised research programme - In the longer term the best prospects for reducing death rates in those who develop cancer is through better organised and co-ordinated, good quality research.

A better organised information system - To replace the current, piecemeal arrangements that are inadequate for operational management (contracts), planning and research (see section 5.3 and Appendix 4).

5.1   KEY AREAS FOR AN IMPROVED SERVICE

5.1.1 A Charter for Cancer Patients

Cancer services are unavoidably complicated and many people, when faced with needing them, are poorly placed to understand what they can reasonably expect. A number of organisations have produced charters for cancer patients covering different aspects of care.

The Review Group believes that these should be brought together into a National Charter which gives cancer patients, their families and local Health Authorities a clear and complete picture of what should be provided from the various parts of the cancer service. Two study groups working on behalf of the Review Group have identified areas which might be incorporated in a charter. We recommend that a small working party comprising representatives of patients, voluntary patient support organisations, the professions, CHCs, provider units and local Health Authorities should be set up to develop this work, within six months.

5.1.2 Access to Services

Certain sections of the population - for example people from ethnic minorities, those with sensory or other disabilities, elderly people - may have special difficulty accessing health and support services. This is particularly true in a multi-cultural metropolis such as London. Local Health Authorities and service providers should take active measures to ensure equitable access - including the provision of interpreting and advocacy services, information in a range of languages and sensitivity to cultural beliefs and customs.

5.1.3 'Health of the Nation' - An increased role for primary care and also for cancer centres.

The DoH has supported **'Europe against Cancer'** since its inception in 1985. It sets a target to reduce cancer deaths by 15% by the year 2000.

In **'Health of the Nation'** (1992) and its associated key area handbook - **'Cancers'** (1993), more specific action is proposed against cancer. This includes the targets set out in the table below, against which we have noted relevant trends in London and the south east.

Health of the Nation Targets	Incidence Trends (From provisional figures provided by the Thames Cancer Registry)
I. Reduce lung cancer deaths in over 75s by at least 30% in men and 15% in women by the year 2010.	Projected 30% increase in women during the 1990s. There is an anticipated roughly equivalent decrease in men. The survival rate from lung cancer is only 5% at 5 years. 80% of the incidence is associated with smoking.
2. Reduce breast cancer in the screened population by at least 25% by the year 2000.	Projected to increase by 7% during the 1990s. Survival rate is between 25% and 50% at 5 years. None of the Thames Regions has achieved the 70% target for breast screening. In some inner London districts uptake is as low as 20%.
3. Cervical cancer to be reduced by at least 20% by the year 2000.	The Thames Regions have amongst the lowest rates in the country, but also have amongst the worst uptake rates for screening. Between a quarter and half of women aged 24-64 in London seem likely to not have been screened for cervical cancer in the last five and half years.
4. Halt the increased incidence of skin cancer by the year 2005.	This is projected to increase by 70% over the 10 years to year 2000. Avoidance and prompt treatment are vital.

The Steering Group supports the initiative of Health of the Nation very strongly. Whilst much of the action it proposes is in primary care, which is not the main subject of this Review, we wish, nevertheless, to underline its fundamental importance.

Specific action to support Health of the Nation Targets

(i)   There is a particular need in London to improve the accuracy of FHSA registration data and target action towards low uptake of screening.

(ii)   The early detection and diagnosis of cancer also requires the prompt investigation of suspicious symptoms. Continuing education programmes for G.P.s and nurses should include sessions on the diagnosis of cancer. The Royal College of General Practitioners should take a lead in developing this in conjunction with the Royal College of Nursing and with relevant specialist involvement from the other medical Royal Colleges.

(iii)   Secondary and tertiary cancer services have an important part to play in supporting the Health of the Nation initiative:

- By acting as a resource for cancer information they can help those working in primary and community care in their task of public education in prevention and early diagnosis. They can also achieve this through example by their staff (such as no smoking policies) and through direct advice to patients and relatives.

- Staff working in other departments in hospitals can act similarly - for instance, in advice to expectant mothers on smoking and on breast and cervical screening.

- Health of the Nation and its Cancer Handbook also stress the importance of good standards of secondary and tertiary services for patients who do develop cancer. Without these, earlier diagnosis holds no benefit. We believe that our proposals for cancer centres will achieve this.

- The Cancer handbook also makes clear the need for rapid access to hospital diagnostic and treatment services for cancer patients. We strongly concur, and believe that the initiative of the Royal Colleges of Physicians and Radiologists in proposing targets in this area ('Quality Control in cancer care: Setting some targets' 1992) should be supported and extended. A fast track system, operated by some hospitals for patients in whom a cancer diagnosis is suspected, and 'one-stop clinics' where all necessary tests are carried out at one visit are examples of good service that we have seen, and strongly support.

5.1.4 Support for cancer patients in the community

Accurate and Timely Information

(i)   General Practitioners and Community Nursing Teams require accurate and timely information from hospitals on the diagnosis and treatment of their patients if they are to provide efficient support and care. We recommend that DHAs/FHSAs should set minimum standards for the content and speed of communications, and monitor the quality of information provided. A formally established care plan and discharge policy should be in place. It should also extend to both out-patient appointments and in-patient stays.

Community Support

(ii)   The trend from inpatient hospital care towards the community support of patients with cancer, requires an integrated response from primary and community health care services. The ability of these services to meet the needs of people with cancer, now and in the future, depends on an appropriate level of resources (mainly staffing). A multi-disciplinary team approach is crucial to the care of patients in the community, yet many GPs in London report difficulties in obtaining paramedical services, particularly occupational therapy and physiotherapy. There is a need for district nursing staff to receive training in specific aspects of oncology nursing, and also to be able to access specialist advice and support.

(iii)   It should be an objective for each patient to have a key worker (often a District or Macmillan nurse). Patient-held record cards are being introduced in some districts, and are seen as being a valuable way of improving the co-ordination of services.

Support for Carers

(iv)   The needs of informal carers for support and information should also be recognised and appropriate provision made.

Follow-up

(v)   The arrangements for follow-up are not always clear to patients or their GPs. These should be made explicit in the treatment plan. Health Authorities should monitor treatment plans.

5.1.5 Palliative Care

(i)   All patients with advanced, incurable cancer require good palliative care. Priority should be given to the control of pain and other symptoms, and to psychological support. The goal is the achievement of the best possible quality of life for these patients and their families.
A comprehensive palliative care service comprises in-patient beds, home care, hospital and day care, and access to specialist pain relief services. It involves a multidisciplinary team of nurses, doctors, social workers, physiotherapists, occupational therapists, chaplains and volunteers.

(ii)   The majority of patients would prefer to die in their own homes but in London over 50% die in hospital. The provision of more domiciliary nursing, if necessary for 24 hours a day, would enable more people to die at home without placing undue strain on relatives and carers.

(iii)   We recommend that Health Authorities should review their palliative care services with a view to improving them, particularly for patients who wish to remain at home. They should develop better integration of the provider units and facilitate co-operation between the various agencies, NHS and voluntary services.

5.1.6 Death and Bereavement

(i)   DHAs/FHSAs should set standards for bereavement support for the families of cancer patients. These should include the provision of written information (on both practical and emotional aspects of bereavement), notification of all relevant agencies, sensitive and flexible arrangements for the collection of personal belongings and equipment, as well as sensitivity to cultural beliefs. A key worker should be nominated to maintain contact with the family during the first 3-6 months of bereavement, and assess any need for more specialist bereavement support.

5.2   IMPROVING LOCAL HOSPITAL SERVICES FOR CANCER PATIENTS

As 70% of people with cancer are 60 years old or more, many find travelling large distances difficult, and may well have other health or social problems; it is important therefore that as much care as possible is provided locally, with outreach specialist support where necessary.

Already some 55% of people diagnosed as having cancer are initially treated in their local general hospital rather than a specialist Centre; we make a number of recommendations to improve this predominant element of the service.

5.2.1 A stronger role for cancer specialists in local acute hospitals

(i)   Nearly half the local acute hospitals which have cancer input have a presence of less than two consultant cancer specialist sessions per week.

(ii)   As noted earlier, the relationships between DGHs and large Cancer Centres have largely been set up on an ad-hoc basis. The amount of consultant oncologist input varies widely:

18%   DGHs have 4 or more Consultant Oncologist sessions per week
18%   DGHs have 3-4 Consultant sessions per week
20%   DGHs have 2-2.75 Consultant sessions per week
31%   DGHs have 1-2 Consultant sessions per week
12%   DGHs have less than one session per week

<u>Too little access to a specialist oncologist's expertise</u>

(iii)   A consequence of this low level of specialist oncology input at District General Hospital level is that too few patients currently have the benefit of a consultant oncologist's opinion or a co-ordinated treatment plan involving, where appropriate, the four main modalities - surgery, oncology, radiotherapy and palliative care. The increasing use of such complex treatment reinforces the need for cancer specialists to spend more time in local hospitals in the future.

<u>Access to specialist nursing support</u>

(iv)   Patients at local acute hospitals should receive nursing support from nurses who have been trained in the care of people with cancer, and have access to a full range of specialist support services.

<u>Standard setting</u>

(v)   The Review recommends that Specialist Cancer Centres should have a leadership role in improving cancer services overall, working in conjunction with other providers within the NHS and those in the voluntary sector. We recommend that local Health Authorities should work with the Specialist Cancer Centres to ensure better co-ordinated local services are introduced, as quickly as possible, and be subject to systematic clinical, managerial and consumer audits.

<u>Spending more time in local acute hospitals</u>

(vi)   The model we recommend for an average-sized local acute hospital (DGH) is that consultant cancer specialists should be available on site for most days of the working week, and on call for urgent consultation. Any one clinical or medical oncologist must however spend enough time at base for continuity of care, and should not in our view spend more than a maximum of four sessions per week at a local acute hospital. (Only 18% of local acute hospitals surveyed currently benefit from this level of specialist input). Smaller acute hospitals may need rather less of an oncology 'on-site' presence; large teaching hospitals that are not tertiary Cancer Centres, considerably more, including good on-site medical oncology facilities in many cases.

<u>A wider role for cancer specialists</u>

(vii)   The wider role to be fulfilled by cancer centre specialists within associated local acute hospitals would be:-

-     Holding joint clinics and ward rounds.

-     Co-ordinating the production of protocols, of more systematic audit across a number of DGHs and higher levels of participation in clinical trials.

- Regularly participating in the postgraduate training programme of the DGH, not least in providing sessions for GPs to keep up to date with information on early diagnosis, treatment options and developments in co-ordinated care (as set out above).

5.2.2 Better organisation of cancer surgery in local acute hospitals (DGH's)

In the past, cancer surgery in local acute hospitals has been under-recognised, being only one of many aspects of the general services. More recently however there has been a trend towards specialisation by individual surgeons in local acute hospitals. The national screening programme has given a particular impetus to improving the quality of breast cancer treatment

During the Review we have sought the views of the Royal College of Surgeons. This has confirmed that greater specialisation should be applied to the care of many cancers, common and less common. Areas besides breast cancer, where surgical specialisation is appropriate are colo-rectal and oesophageal cancer, reconstructive head and neck surgery and urological malignancies. Not only should DGH staff specialise and group themselves in this way, but such groupings should have close, regular and established contacts with tertiary centres and their staff.

Similarly, the Royal College of Obstetricians and Gynaecologists has emphasised the desirability of major surgery for gynaecological cancers being carried out by a greater degree of specialisation.

Section 6.6 gives further details of the arrangements the Review has concluded will improve the surgical management of cancer patients.

5.3   A BETTER ORGANISED RESEARCH PROGRAMME

Cancer research has a strong reputation in London. This includes both basic science research, clinical trials of new methods for diagnosis and treatment, and the uptake of proven developments in practice. In looking forward over the next 10-15 years, we have taken the advice of many research workers, and of those in all the centres we have visited, in order to help us form a view on how best the service arrangements for cancer can support research and development. We believe it to be essential that they should do so effectively, for the benefit of future patients. The views expressed in the following paragraphs represent, we believe, a reasonable distillation of the views expressed to the Review Group.

5.3.1 Epidemiological Research

Cancer research will need to continue to address the whole field of the epidemiology of cancer, where it has had substantial past success (Doll, W.R.S. "Are we winning the war against cancer?" - Keith Durrant Memorial Lecture, 1991).

It will need to study risk factors and prevention, as well as the effectiveness of treatment and rehabilitation. Good and effective working relationships are needed here between clinicians and epidemiologists working in public health medicine, both locally and nationally. Generally, however, this aspect of cancer research does not require to be on-site in a cancer centre. Its effective links with cancer registry data are however of importance.

5.3.2 Basic Science Research

Whilst there may be some advantages in close physical proximity between basic science as it relates to cancer, and hospital-based research and services, these are not strong enough to make single site working essential. Indeed there are examples of 'stand alone' basic science cancer research units in London - such as that of ICRF in Lincoln's Inn Fields which has an excellent track record of good research. Sometimes, however, there will be significant benefits from co-locating basic oncological science with broadly based general science and biological research units of London University, or with basic science relevant to a wide range of medical specialties as is the model at RPMS at Hammersmith Hospital.

Developments in cell biology and molecular genetics hold enormous potential for improving cancer prevention and treatment in the future. They require a concentration of research funding and expertise, and have implications for many other conditions than just cancer. Whilst they require good clinical links, they have we believe the greater need for the close general science and general medicine links proposed above for basic physics, chemistry and other biological research relating to cancer.

5.3.3 New drug and radiation physics development in cancer treatment

New drug development requires a somewhat closer conjunction between the clinic and the laboratory, than does basic science research. Here, however, research also needs close links with animal facilities, as well as those for chemistry and pharmacology. A relatively small hospital presence (providing basic facilities for sample collection) linked to an off-site laboratory base should we believe prove to be only marginally less effective and productive than same-site operation.

The same argument and conclusion does we believe apply to research in radiation physics, although shortage of staff with the required skills may require single site operation to be the practical pattern.

5.3.4 Clinical trials in cancer

Much of the progress in the treatment of cancer that has been achieved in recent years, has only been possible as a result of well organised clinical trials. In these, potential new advances have to be compared with existing methods in a large enough group of patients to establish whether any supposed benefit is real. Despite the promise of some fields of basic cancer research, there is no sign as yet of the development of any new treatment so effective that testing by this means will be unnecessary (c.f. Penicillin, 1941).

All phases of cancer trials necessarily take place based upon the hospital and community services where patients are treated. Usually, the coordination of trials will usefully be carried on from clinical trials offices close to the hospital work place. Some larger multi-centre trials, however, may be operated from a separate site successfully, provided that it is properly staffed and equipped with modern and effective communications. Many multi-centre and international cancer trials have been and are being run effectively in this way. A variation which is sometimes needed is to develop 'satellite' clinical trials offices in cancer centres linked to 'stand alone' national trials centres.

As a large number of patients are needed in most cancer trials to demonstrate any health gain (or lack of it) within a reasonable short time scale, and given the relatively slow natural history of most cancers, it is essential that the greatest possible number of cancer patients be asked to participate in properly designed, peer reviewed trials of new treatments, which has, of course, had Ethical Committee approval. In London, therefore, with its large population, there is a special opportunity to bring together a sufficient number of patients with like conditions, and a strong mix of oncological specialists backed by a broad spread of general hospital groups, so that good quality clinical research can take place. This opportunity, which we believe to be of the greatest importance for cancer patients of the future, will however be lost if the expertise is diluted in many small cancer centres.

Furthermore, benefits derived through clinical cancer research will be more effectively spread and developed in the NHS if backed by careful, peer reviewed research at centres of acknowledged standing, than if many small centres, without a sufficient well-found research base, attempt this task.

5.3.5 Conclusion

We recommend, from evidence submitted to us, that:-

-       Basic cancer research should have its essential links on-site with either university-based science or strong interdisciplinary sciences now established in some hospitals. (Close physical proximity to clinical facilities has some advantages, but is of lower priority).

-       The same should apply, in general, to most biological, molecular genetics and physics research in cancer.

-       New drug development research needs links primarily to laboratory and animal facilities. It also needs however, effective interdisciplinary discussion and communication with clinical services where new drugs are first used, and their benefits and disadvantages first assessed.

- Clinical cancer trials need to be able to involve as large a number of patients as possible. Whilst their technical coordination does not always require a hospital base, close association of specialist oncologists and a broad base of general hospital services should underpin them whenever possible. They should incorporate patients in local acute hospitals by outreach from the interdisciplinary cancer centres.

- Epidemiological cancer research is important. It does not require an on-site hospital base, but clinical and cancer registry links between clinicians and epidemiologists are needed.

5.3.6 Overview of cancer research in London

We have not been able, within the timescale or the remit of our work, to analyze cancer research at the centres in London in any depth. We have however carefully considered the conclusions of the University Selectivity exercise. We have discussed their clinical research plans with all of the units we have visited. We have also had some discussions with senior officers of the Medical Research Council, the Imperial Cancer Research Fund, and the Cancer Research Campaign, and with the NHS Director of Research and Development. Towards the end of our work, we have had some preliminary views from the DoH Research and Development Directorate's SHA research reviews of the Hammersmith and Royal Marsden Hospital Special Health Authorities. We believe that Cancer research could benefit from more detailed study, and we strongly support this as a target for a future NHS R & D initiative.

Combining the information thus gathered, and especially looking forward to the future for cancer research, we have come to some views on how cancer research is likely to be best supported in relation to the service realignments that we believe should be made. These are dealt with generally above, and on a site by site basis in Section 7 of this report.

5.4   A BETTER ORGANISED INFORMATION SYSTEM

5.4.1 Un-coordinated systems

We have previously noted the difficulties caused by the dissociation of the Cancer Registry and Cancer Centre information. Although the recent circular EL(92)95 will improve some parts of cancer registration data, the provision of accurate information on the use of resources by cancer patients will still be inadequate for operational management and planning.

5.4.2 Under-recording

The Cancer Registry data, being population based, only records types of treatment within the first 6 months of registration, and this is only a very approximate estimate of the resources consumed. The information from hospitals does capture information on the resources used, but because it is not yet patient based, is very difficult to link to specific populations, tumour types or individuals, and cannot be checked back properly to the Cancer Registry. Patient-based data from cancer centres has been difficult to relate to Cancer Registry data.

There is probably some undercounting in the Cancer Registry, particularly in the estimates of the proportion of patients who receive radiotherapy and chemotherapy. However there is equally probably substantial double counting in the cancer centre statistics.

These uncertainties have caused us considerable debate about the appropriate treatment workload arising from a defined population. We address these issues in Appendix 4, and make recommendations that we believe are urgent, to address these problems.

5.4.3 New arrangements for information systems

The Review Group recommends that urgent steps need to be taken to:

- Enable linkage of treatment data from providers (including Cancer Centres) to Cancer Registries.

- Develop ways of grouping patients to predict their likely resource use.

This should lead to a system in which the resources used by each person registered with cancer would be captured, enabling monitoring of local treatment and provision of accurate comparative rates.

5.4.4 A Task Group to devise a new system by April 1994

Whether such a system should be a routine, or provide ad-hoc sampling needs to be considered and a cost justified proposals developed. The Review Group recommends that a task group should be set up to develop detailed proposals by April 1994 with implementation, after some market testing, being no later than April 1995. This group should be convened by the Information Management Group and include representatives of the relevant Royal Colleges, National Casemix Office, National Steering Group on Cancer Registration and Health Authorities. This matter, and some other particular problems we encountered, are developed further in Appendix 4.

SECTION 6. THE ORGANISATION OF SPECIALIST CANCER CENTRES WITHIN A METROPOLITAN AREA

6.1 THE PROBLEMS OF EXISTING SMALL SPECIALIST CANCER CENTRES IN LONDON

As previously described the Specialist Cancer Centres in London each treat on average, half the number of new clinical/medical oncology patients treated by the large Metropolitan Centres elsewhere in the U.K. This is a product of history and not justified by the relatively good access times in the South East compared with the rest of the U.K., which reflects the relatively short travel distances and well developed public transport arrangements that exist.

6.1.1 Shortcomings of the small units

The current pattern of l5 small units in London has substantial shortcomings:-

- Unnecessary duplication of buildings and expensive equipment in central London units, leading to poor cost-effectiveness.

- A number of centres have too few consultants to allow them to sub-specialise and keep at the forefront of the management of particular cancers.

- Many of the London Units have difficulty in recruiting staff, especially therapy radiographers and radiation physicists. The present arrangements maximise the requirement for these and other staff.

- The capital investment has hitherto been spread thinly so that many of the existing smallish centres, both within and outside the M25, have an incomplete and/or outdated range of equipment.

- In smaller centres with only one or two linear accelerators (for instance) equipment breakdowns and routine maintenance disproportionately disrupt and often delay treatment.

- Participation by small London centres in research and clinical trials tends to be lower.

- Small departments may lack dedicated porters, and clerical and other support staff, which again impairs the smooth running of the department and makes it less user friendly.

Most of the shortcomings are avoided in larger centres, which also have other advantages set out elsewhere in this report. The Review Group has therefore concluded that, quite apart from the need for there to be a smaller number of hospitals overall in Central London, there is an overwhelming case for creating a smaller number of larger, more comprehensive cancer centres to serve Londoners and others living in the South East.

6.2 THE PLACE OF SPECIALIST CANCER CENTRES WITHIN THE INTERNAL MARKET

Instead of the current 15, the Review proposes that there should be a reduced number of specialist Cancer Centres within the M25. Even this lesser number will however permit a greater level of competition than in any other part of the U.K. By creating a smaller number of more comprehensive Centres, it will be possible for Health Authorities, by collaborative reviews, to more effectively compare performance both in quality and price terms. The local Health Authorities and RHAs consulted during the course of the Review, have emphasised that they would expect to obtain a higher quality service from a smaller number of centres, particularly through better co-ordinated care with local acute hospitals.

The Review Group envisage that the proposed Centres would have the range of staff and facilities to compete in terms of the quality of service they provide, in a way that, from numerous visits made during the course of this study, is not happening at present. It must be stressed again however that much better information will need to be available than at present if competition is to be based, as it should be, on a comparison of like with like.

6.3 ACCESS TO SPECIALIST CANCER SERVICES

(i)   Advice from individual patients and from the national Cancer Patients Support Groups, has confirmed that people with cancer are willing to travel to obtain the best possible treatment. However a main objective of the proposals made in this Review is that as much of the service as possible should be delivered locally, as far as is compatible with good quality, treatment and care. This is particularly important for palliative care. There are two special factors supporting the case for maximising local services for cancer patients:-

-    The majority of patients receiving cancer treatment are elderly.

-    Unlike many other treatments, cancer treatment often involves repeated visits to a specialist centre over several weeks, months or years.

(ii)   We have adopted in our analysis of site options the criterion that 95% of patients should be able to reach a Specialist Cancer Centre within one hour's travel time. Many of the patients treated at centres in other parts of the country have to accept considerably longer travel times.

(iii)   The existing Specialist Cancer Centres vary widely in the extent that they have taken steps to help the patients deal with travelling problems. We recommend that some of the innovative schemes we have seen, should be adopted more generally.

(iv)   The particular measures on which Health Authorities should assess progress by Trust Hospitals are:-

-    Reducing the proportion of patients being brought in groups by ambulance, replacing this arrangement by more individualised transport services.

-    Making adequate provision within overall site constraints for car parking for cancer patients. Cancer outpatients attending frequently for radiotherapy or chemotherapy should not be charged for car parking, in our view.

-    The working hours during which cancer treatment operates should be reviewed to give maximum flexibility for patients. Surveys elsewhere have shown that many prefer early morning or evening treatment.

-    Hotel (warden controlled) and hostel (minimal nursing staff levels) beds should be introduced for those patients who cannot reasonably travel.

6.4   ASSESSING THE APPROPRIATE SIZE OF FUTURE CENTRES

Two or Three Large Centres for London

(i)   The South East is a densely populated area with relatively good travel links, so there is a case for Specialist Cancer Units being larger than in other Metropolitan Centres. The Review Team's assessment is that there are a number of clear advantages in large Centres, in terms of effective use of resources. At the top end of the scale is the Christie Hospital, Manchester, with 10,000 new oncology patients per year. This hospital runs effectively, and its patients and local population support it strongly. It is regarded as a caring hospital, where the views of the individual patient matter.

(ii)   Such a radical approach for London would mean as few as two or three Centres, instead of the existing 15. To achieve this would however require a very high of capital investment. Cancer Centres of this size would be difficult to accommodate within a number of existing acute hospitals in London. Such a small number of centres would each need to be associated with a very large number of both teaching hospitals and local acute Hospitals. This would in our view increase the difficulties of developing the new, proposed level of closer working links.

<u>An efficient size of unit for London</u>

(iii)   Taking into account all it has seen and heard, therefore, the Review Team
         recommends the creation of Centres that are capable of treating some
         3,000 - 4,500 new non-surgical oncology patients per year. Such Units
         would be able to provide a comprehensive specialist cancer service in
         terms of the range of staff expertise, range of equipment, teaching
         potential and effectiveness of the research base. This would mean that
         the new Centres would be two to three times larger on average than
         those that exist across London at present. The proposed Centre would of
         course have associated with an appropriate balance of surgical services
         and all the other supporting services necessary.

(iv)   The Mount Vernon Centre already treats in the region of 4,000 new
         oncology cases per annum, and along with the evidence from even larger
         Centres elsewhere in the U.K., we are confident that units of at least the
         size we propose will be able in the future to provide better quality
         services than currently exist.

(v)   This plan to concentrate specialist cancer services into a number of larger
         units follows the pattern advocated by the International Commission on
         Radiological Protection in its report "Protection of the Patient in Radiation
         Therapy" (ICRP publication no. 44, 1984). This size of unit has been
         supported by advice we have taken from the directors of other cancer
         centres in the U.K. and abroad.

6.5   THE PROPOSED MODEL FOR LONDON

6.5.1 Size

We set out in this section our proposals concerning the levels of staffing
and facilities required for a Centre treating 3,000 new non-surgical
oncology patients per annum (including those seen in linked local
hospitals). They would need to be scaled up for larger units of course,
but not necessarily pro-rata in all respects. There are economies of scale
at least up to the size of 4,500 cases per year. It must be remembered,
however, that linear accelerators come in whole numbers.

6.5.2 Staff

<u>8 Clinical and Medical Oncology Consultants</u> (i.e. excluding surgeons and
haematologists). This will allow greater tumour-specific specialisation,
more effective clinical management of the department, research co-
ordination, and each consultant to spend up to two days per week in a
linked local acute hospital. The proportion of medical oncologists will be
dependent on case-mix and research activities. One palliative care
consultant would also be included in this total. These staffing members
assume the usual present balance of junior medical staff, and the
contribution they make to most service needs. If their numbers or their
service commitments are reduced, additional consultants will be required.

We also assume in these numbers that improved secretarial and administrative backup is provided to free medical staff more than at present for work they alone can undertake.

Radiographers - Such a Centre would require 30-35 posts.

Physicists - The unit would require four to six physicists supported by dedicated physics technicians and engineering support staff.

Pharmacists - The Centre would have two dedicated pharmacists.

Nurses - There should be a range of specialist nurses including those trained and skilled in breast care, palliative care and symptom control, counselling, and tumour site specific expertise, as appropriate. Chemotherapy units should be staffed by nurses with specialist training in intravenous and cytotoxic drug therapy. Such staff would act as an expert resource for the Primary Health Care Team, as well as colleagues in local acute Hospitals. (In-patients would need to be supported by sufficient numbers of qualified nursing staff with post-basic experience and expertise. Grade mix and skill mix would be determined by the dependency levels of the patients, see section on Beds below).

Support Staff - The Centre would require a range of professional staff, especially in the fields of medical social work, physiotherapy, speech therapy, dietetics, occupational therapy, and particularly for London, an interpretation service. It would also of course require well trained reception, administration and clerical staff. There would need to be appropriate electronic and mechanical engineering staff and equipment, to the planned degree of in-house equipment maintenance. Suitable arrangements would need to be in place for liaison with pathology services, especially routine and urgent haematology and chemical pathology. Similarly effective coordination with Imaging Departments is important.

6.5.3 Radiotherapy Equipment

5 Linear Accelerators - One with a high energy capacity and two capable of providing electrons. Such a Centre should also have a spare bunker so machine replacements can be achieved without major service disruption and expansion is allowed for. Based on model throughput and machine utilisation rates, the number of Linacs required falls between four and five. However, to allow for future growth in patient numbers and possible variations in the referral patterns projected, the higher number has been used in our projections.

2 Simulators the trend towards Centres of this size having a CT/simulator will reduce somewhat the reliance on imaging equipment outside the department. This will also shorten the time it takes to prepare a radiation treatment plan and reduce the attendances that a patient needs to make before starting treatment. One of the two simulators

should therefore probably be of this type. Some savings in staff time are likely to also result.

<u>2 Treatment Planning Computer Systems</u>

<u>2 Brachy Therapy Units</u> (high or low dose-rate)

<u>1 Superficial X-ray Treatment Machine</u>

6.5.4 Beds

Although there is likely to be a variation between units, the figure of some 50-60 beds (excluding the needs of surgical patients), is seen as a reasonable number, on the assumption that:-

- 10% will be hotel beds i.e. unstaffed usually double rooms, allowing patients who find travelling difficult to be accommodated with a carer.

- 20% will be hostel beds i.e. with a relatively low level of on-site day time nursing support.

- 20% of the beds will be operated on a five day basis i.e. be closed at weekends.

- Of the remaining 50%, the majority will need to be staffed for the dependency levels found in typical acute medical ward, with a declining proportion of beds being for palliative care as further community provision is made. In centres where very intensive chemotherapy is given, and for bone marrow transplantation, special in-patient facilities are needed (see section 6.8).

This number is dependent on effective links with local acute hospitals also existing, so that cancer patients would have their hospital care locally where appropriate.

It is assumed that units would provide, in addition, up to l0 couches/beds for chemotherapy carried out on a day-case basis, as well as for blood transfusions.

We recommend that the bed numbers be reviewed periodically in the light of the trend towards more day care as against the growing number of elderly people with multi-system disease needing inpatient care.

6.5.5 Chemotherapy Facilities

Proper facilities will be required for safe cytotoxic drug preparation, staffed usually by pharmacists. Chemotherapy patients will often now be able to receive their treatment in day care units which will require some specialised chairs, beds and other equipment.

6.5.6 Haemato-oncology facilities

Described separately - see section 6.8.

6.6 SHOULD CANCER CENTRES STAND ALONE OR BE SET IN GENERAL HOSPITALS WITH OTHER SPECIALIST SERVICES?

6.6.1 The historic pattern

It has been put to the Review Group that at least one Cancer Centre in London should be of sufficient size that it can properly support all the services needed, to stand alone as a tertiary centre for the diagnosis and treatment of cancer, and with special expertise in teaching and cancer research. There are American models for this, such as the M.D. Anderson Hospital in Houston and the Memorial Hospital in New York. There are also Cancer Centres in the U.K. which by chance more than by planning, are in hospitals which do not have a full range of general services. Examples are Clatterbridge Hospital, (Liverpool), Cookridge Hospital, (Leeds), and also the Christie Hospital, (Manchester). In London, the Royal Marsden was established and has functioned in this way, in recent years, on its two sites. At the time the Royal Marsden was founded, 150 years ago, there was a real need to understand and to treat cancer better, and to concentrate expertise and research in such a way was wholly appropriate.

6.6.2 The limitations for the future of stand-alone cancer centres

(i)   Since this is a most important matter of principle, we have consulted very widely with experts in many facets of the care and management of hospital and cancer services, and with senior medical and cancer research workers. We have also asked this question of all of the groups and service leaders we have seen and visited in London.

(ii)   Our conclusion is that this is not the pattern of care that should be the preferred model for the future, for the following reasons:

-       Cancer services are concerned with the care of acutely ill patients, for whom direct access, on site, to general and specialist physicians and surgeons is very desirable. Most cancer patients are older people needing a wide range of other expertise from medical and paramedical staff, as do other elderly patients.

-       The general diagnostic and support services for cancer, such as pathology and imaging, are required just as much for patients who do not have cancer, as for those who do. Duplication of such expensive services is quite wrong in both equipment and manpower terms. Equally, it is desirable that the specialists who work in this field should maintain a breadth of diagnostic expertise from a mix of medical cases, which should not and does not prevent their own development of special interests in cancers or in other fields.

- New developments in radiotherapy equipment, for instance, multi-leaf collimators are now already being tested in several Centres in the U.K. This dispersed pattern of innovation has we believe been a strength of the NHS. There seems no special reason why such testing should in future be restricted to any one Centre, which would not necessarily have the expertise in its staff for any particular specialised development. This would in any case be against a 'market philosophy', as exemplified by the links which some departments already have which assist manufacturers to develop their equipment in conjunction with, and with benefit for, the N.H.S.

- New developments in molecular medicine and genetics, whilst they strike at the very causes of cancer, and hence hold real hope of advances in prevention and treatment, are also of great significance for many other medical and surgical conditions; inflammatory bowel disease, asthma and diabetes for example. It is, we are advised, essential that these research developments are exploited in association with the research environment of general medical services, not cancer alone.

- Staff in training, whether in medical, paramedical or supporting services do we believe learn best within the broad environment of general acute services, rather than by working wholly in a specialist hospital.

(iii)   None of these features mean that a Cancer Centre that forms part of a general hospital should not have its own identity, targets and philosophy of care and research. We believe it should. There are good examples of this in London and elsewhere now. But we believe that looking ahead, isolated cancer units should relocate their activities to be closely conjoined with general hospital services.

(iv)   In London, this matter mainly concerns the Royal Marsden Hospital. We believe that it can be resolved to a considerable extent by relocation of Fulham Road functions to Sutton, and by the strengthening of already existing clinical links between Sutton and St. George's. But we do not propose that any new cancer centres should be developed in isolation from general hospitals.

6.7 A PROPOSED PATTERN FOR THE CARE OF PATIENTS WITH COMMON, LESS COMMON AND RARER CANCERS, WITH SPECIAL REFERENCE TO SURGERY

6.7.1 Common cancers

These occur with a frequency of greater than a hundred per million people, such as those of the breast, lung, skin, and colo-rectum, and require expertise and facilities for treatment and care in the community and at hospitals at all levels of specialisation. The Royal College of Surgeons believes that these patients should have the advantage of care by a sufficient number of surgeons to allow some specialisation in the treatment of these cancers so that the surgical management of the patient will be carried out by a surgeon with a special interest in each disease. At the same time these local surgical teams will require backup and regular on-site consultation with oncology specialists from the most local cancer centre. Formal joint clinics will be an important part of the liaison which is needed here, but they will not be necessary in all circumstances, nor must patients wait for infrequent joint clinics when clear diagnosis and management decisions are waiting to be taken.

6.7.2 Less common cancers

Cancers which occur with an incidence of say a hundred per million population will, even so, be sufficiently common that not all will be appropriately treated within a special cancer centre. Some of these patients will be suffering from cancers which can be entirely managed on a local basis especially when the treatment available is either relatively uncomplicated or has become standard, or when the disease is so advanced that the skills of palliative care and support are the prime need.

Many of these less common cancers do however require special surgical or non-surgical oncology expertise if the patient is to have the best chance of cure or palliation. Examples would include cancers of the oesophagus, stomach, kidney, bladder, pancreas, liver, thyroid, ovary, cervix, and head and neck cancer. It is impractical for all these patients to be treated within a specialist cancer centre, or even within the general medical and surgical services attached to the centre, but there are advantages in sub-specialisation in their management both at surgical and non-surgical specialist level.

Arrangements should be set up so that in all of the local acute hospitals served by a cancer centre there are clear arrangements for the surgical and non-surgical management of these patients. In some cases this would mean that one or more surgeons across the group of local acute hospitals may develop special expertise so that cross referral should take place. In others one or more surgeons within a local acute hospital may agree to meet the need. In both instances close links with the non surgical services at the cancer centre should be established, either with joint clinic arrangements or in other ways, so that appropriate management is set up and monitored.

6.7.3 Rare cancers

There has been shown to be clear advantage in referring certain rare cancers to very specialised centres and these centres will in London normally be the Tertiary Unit. In some cases formal supra regional services have already been established - for instance in choriocarcinoma at Charing Cross Hospital, the surgical management of patients with primary bone tumours by endo prosthetic replacement at the Middlesex in conjunction with the Royal National Orthopaedic Hospital Trust and the retinoblastoma service at Bart's. In other cases special expertise will have been developed and will continue in one or more tertiary centre to which patients with particular rare tumours will best continue to be referred. Present examples might be the treatment of soft tissue sarcomas in which particular experience has been gained at University College Hospital and at the Royal Marsden Hospital, and in neuro-oncology which would generally need to be located in relation to neurosurgical services.

6.7.4 Progress in research

For rare and less common tumours progress is likely to be best facilitated by the collection of the greatest possible number of patients with a like diagnosis in one place, so that existing treatments can be tested and new ones evaluated in a properly structured way with of course the individual patient's full agreement and consent.

6.8 PATHOLOGY AND IMAGING SERVICES

In the new structure of fewer, larger specialist cancer centres closely linked to major general hospitals, there will we believe generally be available all of the supporting medical services that patients with cancer require for rapid, accurate diagnosis and treatment.

These will include histo and cyto pathology, chemical pathology, the pathology of infections whether by bacteria, viruses or fungal or other agents, immunopathology and other disciplines. The specialist referral centres for histopathology of certain less common cancers should of course be maintained, with their existing cross reference procedures, for which special financial arrangements may be required. There will be a need for special arrangements for haematology, which we cover in the following section.

The treatment of cancer, especially when it is with the hope of care, now requires very careful preliminary assessment of the position and extent of the tumour, in which diagnostic imaging plays a vital part. Modern imaging techniques need all to be available, including conventional and contrast radiology and CT scanning, ultrasound, scinti-scanning with radionuclides, and magnetic resonance imaging which is now providing its worth in tumour localisation. Existing guidelines for the most effective use of these services should be followed, in liaison with the clinical director of radiology services.

6.9 HAEMATOLOGY IN ONCOLOGY SERVICES

6.9.1 Routine Haematology

Departments of Haematology support all the routine haematological requirements for cancer treatment. This back-up may involve considerable workload, including much urgent work and also out-of-hours commitment when immuno-suppressed patients are being intensively treated. Their continuing treatment depends upon frequent monitoring of white cell and platelet counts, and upon specialised techniques and advice in relation to intercurrent infections. Whilst such departments support all local acute and teaching hospitals, they will need to be especially strong where tertiary cancer services are also provided, as will the appropriate microbiology and other pathological services.

6.9.2 Specialist Haematology and Oncology

Haematologists are also responsible for the care and treatment of patients with blood-related malignant disease, primarily leukaemia. In addition, haematologists care for a proportion of patients with malignant lymphomas and myeloma, the proportion varying with local expertise and arrangements. In all these patients, collaboration with radiotherapy is often needed.

Different levels of intensity of care are required for various kinds of 'haematological' malignancy, and the Review Group is advised that these can be broadly divided into four groupings, which help to determine where the care is most appropriately given, as follows:-

6.9.3 Local Acute Hospital Services

These will generally be responsible for the standard treatment for the older age-group patients with acute and chronic leukaemia, myeloma and malignant lymphomas - often in liaison with visiting clinical oncology services and with General Practitioners.

6.9.4 More complex Local Acute Hospital Care

In many of the larger local acute hospitals which do not work as tertiary cancer centres, there will be a need for haematologists who have special expertise and back-up to undertake the more complex high dose treatments required for young patients with acute leukaemia, and some related conditions which are now generally managed by reasonably standard protocols.

There will be a requirement here for some in-patient beds. Such centres will require good general laboratory back-up especially in micro-biology, and immuno phenotyping. They may carry out autologous (same patient) bone marrow transplants supported by peripheral stem cell harvest and the use of growth factors. Since induction is mainly by chemotherapy, on-site radiotherapy is not required. A critical mass of experience is however needed for autologous BMT, and we are advised, and recommend, that no centre should offer this service unless at least ten such transplants are carried out per year. These patients require a single room, reverse barrier nursing and positive pressure filtered air.

6.9.5 Tertiary Level

Here it is necessary to have available all of the required facilities for allogenic (sibling) bone marrow transplants, for haematological malignancy, and for some solid tumours. Much of this work is as yet mainly applicable only to children and young adults, and such services should, therefore, be based where those for paediatric or adolescent oncology are provided. These services will require all the support for marrow or peripheral stem cell collection and storage, which may well include marrow culture - therefore significant laboratory back-up is needed. This should include cytogenetics and molecular biology. They will also need in-patient facilities, including reverse barrier nursing and positive pressure, filtered ventilation.

Generally, such centres will be in hospitals which are tertiary Cancer Centres, with on-site radiotherapy, a full clinical oncology back-up, and a range of general medical services needed in support of such patients. They will also provide a focus for training of staff, and for research and development.

6.9.6 Special Referral Level

Those Centres leading development in haematology will provide services for certain special categories of patients where particular developing techniques, usually in clinical trials, are being investigated before routine application. At present, bone marrow transplantation in unrelated matched donors would come within this group, as would treatments now being developed for chronic myeloid leukaemia. Such centres will generally also provide secondary and tertiary services. They will require on-site radiotherapy.

It needs to be remembered that the value and place of BMT in unrelated donors for common solid tumours has not yet been established by clinical trials, so that the service needs cannot yet be determined, nor should this service be routinely available until its value is definitely known.

6.9.7 Conclusions from the Site Visits are as follows:

- That a substantial amount of investment, much of it using charitably donated funds, has been made in many Centres to create specialised facilities to treat patients with blood-related malignancies.

- That overall the number of centres offering a quite specialised range of facilities that now exist in the London hospitals appears greater than can be justified by the current or projected demand for these services in specialist centres, using the criteria for levels of complexity set out above.

- That the trend towards further development of these services in local acute hospitals, is likely to increase the potential over-capacity in specialist centres.

- That London Centres will probably not continue in the future to carry out over 50% of all U.K. bone marrow transplants which they do now.

- We make a recommendation to resolve these problems in Section 7.7.

SECTION 7. EVALUATION OF SITE OPTIONS FOR THE ELEVEN EXISTING INNER LONDON CENTRES

7.1 REFERRAL PATTERNS

7.1.1 Referral to cancer centres in the South East

94% of patients attending the 21 Specialist Centres in the South East live within the four Thames Regions. The biggest inflow is from the Oxford Region, some 1200 new clinical/medical oncology patients per annum (75% of the total). We have assumed that this will reverse over the next five years by 50%, which may even be an underestimation given the developing Oxford Region units. This will affect the West London Quadrant particularly, notably the Charing Cross, Hammersmith and the Royal Marsden (Fulham) and Mount Vernon Hospitals.

7.1.2 Future referral patterns to London cancer centres

The Internal Market

Looking at trends in referral patterns that already exist, based on access and apparent cost differentials. Several conclusions are possible even at this early stage of the NHS reforms:-

- More patients living in and near London will wish to receive as much of their treatment as they can, as locally as possible.

- They will tend to use their nearest tertiary cancer centre in access terms, subject to it providing a good general range of services with the expectation of good care and outcome.

- Health Authorities and G.P.'s will reflect these factors in their contracts/referral patterns.

- Cancer centres part of whom present catchment area is (for historical reasons) very distant will tend to lose this to a more accessible centre. This will have effects which are difficult to analyze and predict in detail, especially to the north and west of London. Our proposals for the North Middlesex, Royal Free, UCH/Middlesex, Hammersmith and Mount Vernon hospitals, have sought to forecast the future pattern, but using comparative price or future quality rather than access may through the internal market produce a different profile.

The effect of these factors could make some of these centres larger than we have proposed (all are able to accommodate moderate enlargement) but as a result reduce the size of others and so risk their viability.

-58-

In making our proposals we have assumed that of the 14.2M living in the Thames Regions, the six centres outside the M25 will in future serve a population of 5.7M by 1996/97, as opposed to 5.1M now. The proposed centres within the M25 therefore require the capacity to care for 8.6M population, allowing for some continuance of patient flows from other Regions.

An allowance has also been made for London centres continuing to provide:-

- The treatment of cancer in children now concentrated at two or three Centres in Central London.

- The treatment of rare cancers in adults which will also predominantly still take place within the smaller number of Centres which we propose within London.

- The development of particular specialist techniques will tend predominantly to be in London Centres.

- With the increase in public awareness, the demand for second opinions will increase and will be met predominantly by London Centres.

The combined effect of these factors will not however be more than marginal in relation to total numbers of patients, who will increasingly seek local care.

7.1.3 Future referral patterns to individual centres

With the trend towards cancer specialists spending a larger portion of their working week in particular local acute hospitals, referral patterns are anticipated as becoming more clearly directed to a particular Cancer Centre, as a consequence of the closer working practices, including joint policies and protocols.

Local Health Authorities which will fund services from the local acute and Specialist Cancer Centres, and also Regional Health Authorities, have strongly supported the proposed pattern of more closely co-ordinated care between groups of local acute hospitals and a particular Specialist Cancer Centre.

7.2 FUTURE DISTRIBUTION OF CANCER CENTRES

7.2.1 Specialist centres outside central London

The Review Group has concluded that it is desirable to retain, and indeed strengthen, the pattern of Specialist Cancer Centres outside the central

London area. These have been discussed in section 8 of the report, which covers North Middlesex, Oldchurch, the Surrey Branch of the Royal Marsden and Mount Vernon Hospitals. That section also gives limited consideration to the six specialist Cancer Centres that lie outside the M25, but still inside the four Thames Regions; namely Colchester, Southend, Canterbury, Maidstone, Brighton and Guildford (with Midhurst) Hospitals, and to the Reading and Northampton Units in Oxford Region.

7.2.2 Inner London centres

Given the populations to be served, the analysis of the options for the future pattern of Specialist Centres has been carried out on the basis of the following four sectors of London, which we have called quadrants:-

- A North Eastern Quadrant, including St. Bartholomew's Hospital and the Royal London Hospital;

- A South Eastern Quadrant, including King's College, Guy's and St. Thomas' Hospitals;

- A South West/Western Quadrant, including the Royal Marsden (Fulham), Charing Cross, St. Mary's and the Hammersmith Hospitals;

- A Northern Quadrant, including the Royal Free and U.C.H./Middlesex Hospitals.

7.2.3 Criteria used in the evaluation of options

Given the number of existing units and the extent of recent capital investment we cannot see a case for any completely new Cancer Centres being built within the M25. We have, therefore, examined the relative suitability of existing sites to take on an expanded role in terms of one assessment of;-

- Their accessibility to an enlarged population which each of the proposed Centres will serve.

- The security of the current and future referral patterns to each unit.

- The range of other specialties anticipated as being on each site.

- The current and anticipated strength of each unit in teaching and research relevant to higher quality cancer services being provided.

- The extent of capital investment required and the quality of the service organisation that is likely to be produced by this, as well as the ease with which further expansion could take place.

The staffing and revenue consequences of our proposals, in so far as the complexity of changes involved, allow judgements to be made.

Each of the quadrants sectors has been examined in turn.

7.3 THE NORTH EAST QUADRANT

7.3.1 Profile of the services provided

NORTH EAST QUADRANT	ROYAL LONDON	ST. BART'S	TOTAL
Total New Clinical Oncology Cases	1,741	1,865	3,606
Total RT Courses	1,915	1,732	3,647
+ Total RT Machines	4 (5)	4 (5)	8 (10)
Total Chemotherapy Doses	7,036	6,590	13,626
*Total Oncology Bed Days	5,261	21,004	26,265
Average Available Onc. Beds	14	72	86
**Income RT	£1,352,000 (est. split)	£873,000	£2,225,000
Chemotherapy	£762,000 (est. split)	£1,226,000	£1,988,000
Haematology & Other	£2,962,000 (est. split)	£2,267,000	£5,229,000
% of the whole hospital revenue income represented by the above (% of whole hospital's capital charges) - shown in brackets	4.5% (6.1%)	2.5% (2.5%)	
Consultant Clinical and Medical Oncology Staff (WTE)	5.0	5.7	10.7

Notes: see overleaf

+   Linear accelerators, cobalt and deep x-ray machines have been used as a proxy for the range of equipment available in 1991/92.

Figures in brackets show current total including any being commissioned.

*   Includes medical and clinical oncology patients
* *   Excluding capital charges

Source: Returns from centres (1991/92 unless otherwise stated).

7.3.2 Referral patterns

Royal London	Bart's
446 (Tower Hamlets) 382 (Newham) 246 (Redbridge) 202 (Barking) 150 (NE Essex) 316 (Other)	607 (City & Hackney) 191 (Bloomsbury & Islington) 149 (Waltham Forest) 118 (Redbridge) 59 (Haringey) 740 (Other)
1741	1865

Both the radiotherapy and medical oncology services of St. Bartholomew's serve a more dispersed population than those of the Royal London Hospital. The St. Bartholomew's catchment is also covered by other units whereas that of the Royal London is more discrete with less competition.

7.3.3 Access

St. Bartholomew's Hospital and the Royal London Hospital are only two and half miles apart. Both have convenient tube stations and a large number of bus routes. St. Bartholomew's is better placed than the Royal London Hospital in terms of the number of nearby mainline stations. Neither hospital has significant on-site car parking. St. Bartholomew's Hospital has some dedicated spaces associated with its Cancer Centre and also has a commercial car park close by, which is being expanded.

The conclusion of the Review Group is that in examining the population that the two centres serve, the public transport links to both sites are well developed and are within the travel limit set for the study. Both hospitals are situated in areas where 'peak hours' traffic congestion is normal and so access times by road are substantially extended during the rush hour compared with off peak periods.

7.3.4 Commitment to a single north east London centre

The two hospitals are working within a single 'shadow' Trust and the Consultants involved in Cancer Services have committed themselves to a single site unit. The Review Team was impressed by the high level of medical leadership apparent at both institutions seeking to create a new identity, unifying the previously separate institutional loyalties. Whilst having the skills, facilities and patient population to offer a comprehensive and excellent spread of cancer services, the proposed North East London Cancer Centre will have particular strengths in pelvic cancers (colo-rectal, gynaecological, urological) as well as neuro-oncological cancers. The Review Team agrees that only one centre for radiotherapy and specialised medical oncology should be provided between the two hospitals, to serve the patients in this quadrant of London.

7.3.5 Assessing the two sites

(i)   This assessment primarily considers the issues relating to cancer services on the two sites and it is hoped it will be a helpful contribution to the full site appraisal which the new Trust intends carrying out.

(ii)   The particular strengths of the St. Bartholomew's centre include:

-       The close unification of its non-surgical oncology services, with high standard clinical and medical oncologists and supporting staff, working together to provide excellent care for patients. The medical oncology unit has substantial ICRF funding, especially relating to paediatric oncology.

-       The high quality children's services involving a wide range of different specialists. This unit treats 100 children a year of whom 25% have retinoblastoma (a Supraregional Service). Close multi-disciplinary working between clinical and medical oncologists, ophthalmic surgeons, anaesthetists and paediatricians is the key to the excellence of this service. The children's accommodation is of good quality and a parents' hostel is on site.

-       Recent capital investment includes a new Haematology ward within one of the main ward blocks, a new theatre suite and new equipment for the radiotherapy department. (This level of recent investment is not atypical of that seen in many centres across London).

(iii)   The advantages of the Royal London Hospital include:-

-       A particularly wide range of regional specialties which, if retained on site as seems likely, would allow a more complete cancer service to be provided than at St. Bartholomew's with surgical and non-surgical specialisation in oncology, and a wide range of local services.

- The Royal London Hospital has a secure, long term future based on serving a substantial local population extending into Essex. It is judged to be a more 'secure market' than that of St. Bartholomew's. Changes proposed elsewhere in this report mean the workload of the Royal London Hospital will increase while that of St. Bartholomew's will reduce.

- The Royal London Hospital also has a large general paediatric service which may be important for the continued development of specialist children's cancer services. (Although as only two or three such centres are recommended by the Paediatric Specialty Review, another site may be recommended).

(iv) The option described in 'Making London Better' of St. Bartholomew's becoming a small specialist hospital has been considered carefully by the Review Group. Our conclusion is that this would not be desirable unless it can be guaranteed that the special services collected together would be offer a very broad range, and with security in the internal market. Otherwise, the cancer service unit would become increasingly isolated and not able to offer a complete service. This option would represent a poor choice given the availability within two and half miles on the Royal London site of the most complete range of specialist services in the capital, including neuro-sciences, plastic surgery, cardiac and renal units, backed by substantial general medical services and support. Furthermore St. Bartholomew's would be likely to lack a comprehensive child health service which we understand is regarded as a pre-requisite for specialist children's services in the future.

(v) Another drawback to centralising specialist cancer services on the St. Bartholomew's site is that key elements of the cancer services are located in different buildings separated by roads. Given site constraints, the major capital investment required to create an enlarged centre would still not result in an integrated unit where wards, radiotherapy department, imaging services, day-care clinics and other services would be closely related to each other, and to general hospital services.

7.3.6 Conclusions

(i) The conclusion of the Review Group is that given the opportunity presented by the exceptionally broad specialty mix already present and anticipated to increase within the Royal London Hospital, and the range of local services based on its large catchment population, this hospital provides the better option in which to site a high quality cancer centre for this part of London for the future.

(ii)   There will be a major managerial task to ensure that the particular areas of medical excellence in some of the specialist cancer services at St. Bartholomew's are transferred intact and without damage.

(iii)   Although the facilities at the Royal London are not as dispersed as those at St. Bartholomew's and an integrated set of services can be created, there would, nevertheless, be a requirement for a capital investment on a scale greater than required in a number of other quadrants in London. A commitment to such a substantial capital scheme of the order of £11M needs to be given, as a matter of priority, if the service to people in this part of London is to match the physical facilities already available in some other quadrants of London. This would be the equivalent of the capital development now in progress at Guildford, but only half the cost of that recently completed at Maidstone. An early decision is also important to prevent the groups of high quality staff based at St. Bartholomew's from breaking up.

(iv)   It has been assumed that, given the scale of investment and the inevitable 'lead time' on the Royal London site that the new Essex Unit will have opened and be of a size and quality that the workload of the Royal London will not attract more than 25% of the patients currently treated at the Oldchurch Unit. The Royal London Unit is therefore expected to serve a population of 1.1m and have sufficient facilities for 3600 new clinical/medical oncology patients per annum, which can be estimated by scaling up our recommendations in 6.4 above.

(v)   We believe that this change has the challenging opportunity of combining the broad patient base and existing skills and service of the Royal London Hospital, the excellent academic track record at St. Bartholomew's centre.

7.4 THE SOUTH EAST QUADRANT

7.4.1 Profile of the services provided

S.E. LONDON	GUY'S	St. Thomas'	KING'S	TOTAL
Total New Clinical Oncology Cases	1,147	1,311	1,088	3,546
Total RT Courses	4,207			4,207
+ Total RT Machines	7			7 (7)
Total Chemotherapy Doses	3,090	1,516	881	5,487
*Total Oncology Bed Days	N/A	N/A	N/A	N/A
Average Available Onc.Beds	36	38	16	90
** Income RT	£4.137M	Included in Guy's	£3.253M	
Chemotherapy	£4.922M	Included in Guy's		
Haematology & Other	£2.036M	Included in Guy's		
% of the whole hospital revenue income represented by the above (% of whole hospital's capital charges)	4.7% (4.1%)	Included in Guy's	2.6% (2.8%)	
Consultant Clinical and Medical Oncology staff (WTE)	10.7			10.7

+ Linear accelerators, cobalt and deep x-ray machines have been used as a proxy for the whole of the range of equipment available in 1992/3.

* Includes medical and clinical oncology cases.

** Excluding capital charges

Source: Returns from centres (1991/92 unless otherwise stated).

7.4.2 Referral Patterns

(No breakdown between sites provided.)

Guy's/King's/Thomas
674 (Bromley)
567 (L & NS)
426 (Camberwell)
390 (Greenwich)
390 (D & G)
1099 (Other)
3546

7.4.3 Access

Guy's and St. Thomas' Hospitals are within one and half miles of each other and King's is only some four miles south at Denmark Hill.

7.4.4 Previous history of creating a single centre

As long ago as 1982 the RHA proposed that the three units at Guy's, King's and St.Thomas's should be merged into a single unit to serve a population of some 1.6m people. The desire of each of the three teaching hospitals, which were at that time separately managed, to retain their own radiotherapy department, prevented this plan being implemented.

However, the problems of the three separate units continued to be apparent and in 1985 unified management arrangements were introduced by the creation of SELRC. This has produced considerable benefits e.g. the 24 pieces of major equipment, much of it outdated, have been replaced with 11 modern machines. By pooling physics and radiography staff for the three sites the potential detrimental effect on patient safety of persistent staff shortage has been minimised.

It is the Review Group's view that the benefits of the unified management arrangements under SELRC have been fully realised, yet the fundamental drawbacks of the current three site arrangements are now even more clear than in the early 1980's.

7.4.5 Problems of the existing arrangements

(i)   The Review Group has serious concerns about the provision of a radiotherapy service split between three sites, and the detrimental effects this has on providing a patient focused service, on patient safety and effective communication with patients and their GPs. Specific areas of concern include:-

-   The absence of radiotherapy simulation equipment on the Guy's and King's sites, and of planning equipment at King's.

-   The incomplete range of treatment equipment at King's and Guy's.

-   The increased likelihood of patient treatment being disrupted by these two sites only having one Linac each, by breakdown or routine maintenance.

(ii) Other adverse consequences for patients of these organisational arrangements are:-

-   That the diagnostic and treatment services they require may make them to attend, for the same condition, two or even all three of the sites.

-   This deprives patients of continuity of staff support. It is the antithesis of patient focused care.

(iii) The drawbacks for staff are:-

-   Significant loss of working time due to travelling between sites.

-   Sessions in local DGHs are fewer than there should be, averaging only one per consultant per week.

-   Effective communication with GPs is hampered by up to three oncology departments and separate surgical units being involved in a patient's care.

-   Organising staff cover is difficult across three sites.

-   The development of specialisation amongst oncologists is inhibited when they cannot work together in one centre.

-   The limited number of radiotherapists/medical oncologists on each site, make integrated working with oncological surgeons more difficult to achieve.

-       The development of audit and systematic development of treatment protocols is held back.

-       Research including involvement in multi-centre cancer trials, is hindered by the lack of a 'critical mass', support services, patients and time.

(iv)   The potential disadvantage of single site operation, namely the loss of a permanent oncologist presence at two of the three sites, would need to be prevented by the development of stronger links between the chosen site, the other two hospitals concerned, and also surrounding DGH's.

(v)   The Oncologists at all three units support the creation of a single site Specialist Cancer Centre to serve South East London, subject to the implementation plan being well organised.

7.4.6 Description of the three current centres

<u>St. Thomas'</u>

St. Thomas' radiotherapy department is the biggest of the three in terms of patients treated; it was reported to us as carrying out 50% of the total workload. (The data provided and checked with the units indicates that it provides a rather smaller proportion). It has the simulation equipment for all three sites and has three megavoltage machines compared with Guy's having two and King's one. The radiography and physics staffing for all three sites is organised from the St. Thomas' department. The Department has the most modern and best designed physical facilities of the three. The St. Thomas' radiotherapy facilities would be the most economical to expand and it would be possible to do so and still retain a coherently grouped set of functions.

The radiotherapy and oncology wards are located in a good quality modern ward block. There are no palliative care beds at present, although there are plans to establish these with the oncology beds. St. Thomas' has the only Academic Department of palliative medicine in the country, a development which we wish to support most strongly. The chemotherapy production facilities are cramped and need to be expanded.

Should St. Thomas' be chosen as the future site for South East London Specialist Cancer Centre, the expanded ward and other accommodation could be grouped to provide a contiguous set of facilities, reasonably close to the expanded Radiotherapy Department.

Guy's

Facilities at Guy's are more dispersed than those on the St. Thomas' site. The new phase of development (£130m) will include exceptionally high quality oncology research areas, day care chemotherapy facilities, and out-patient areas.

Compared with St. Thomas' the Radiotherapy Department has just under half the floor area, is cramped, less modern, and less well appointed. The Radiotherapy Department could be expanded to meet the requirements of the South East London Cancer Centre, but would be less easily achieved and more expensive than the expansion of radiotherapy facilities on the St. Thomas' site, and would still be in a separate area from other parts of the cancer service.

Factors in favour of the Guy's site include the good standing of surgical oncology; for example, the ICRF Breast Unit, which displays a high level of integrated multi-modality care. There has also been a very substantial level of investment in R & D facilities. Guy's has the largest medical oncology unit of the three sites. The chemotherapy inpatient facilities are good although preparation areas are poor. Day care appears relatively under-developed, and the arrangements for the preparation of cytotoxic drugs do not reach required standards.

King's

The Radiotherapy Department was purpose built. It is less cramped than the Guy's department, but has a somewhat outdated appearance and very limited potential for expansion. The facilities for inpatients at the King's site have been modernised to differing extents within the limitations of the 100 year old building.

The haematology unit is in high standard accommodation which includes modern ventilated rooms to minimise the risks of cross infection for immuno-suppressed patients. The unit deals with 180-200 cases of blood-related malignancy per year and is reported to be the largest in the South East Thames Region. It also meets the large demand for treating patients with haemogobinopathies.

The well organised breast screening unit is accommodated in good standard, adapted accommodation. The King's Unit has a relatively large element of its overall workload devoted to treating breast and skin cancers. The Clinical Trials Research Centre is an important resource, as are the links with the Molecular Biology Unit of King's College.

Despite some of these strengths, the current physical facilities for cancer services of King's are, however, the poorest of the three centres and the Unit's representatives agreed that they could not be effectively expanded to provide the high quality facilities needed for the major cancer centre required for South East London. The King's Trust, therefore, acknowledged that its site is unlikely to be the centre for such an enlarged unit although a strong wish was expressed to retain and develop its present medical oncology service. If a complete new build would be required for the South East London Cancer Treatment Centre, then the Trust has identified a potential site and wished this option to be thoroughly examined.

7.4.7 Options for a single centre for South East London

(i)   The Review Group believes that the creation of a single site Specialist Cancer Centre to serve South East London would provide a substantially better service to the people of this part of London than the current disjointed arrangements.

(ii)   In terms of access by road, the three units differ only marginally. However Guy's and St. Thomas' have better public transport links to serve a wider population than King's, given their proximity to main line termini.

(iii)   The King's Unit has suggested that it should be expanded to a two Linac centre, while the Guy's and St. Thomas' units reduce to a single site.

(iv)   Given the better accessibility, the quality of the facilities and the balance, size and research potential of the existing services, the Review Group believes the S.E. London Centre should be located within the Guy's/ St. Thomas' Trust, so avoiding a complete rebuild as would be required on the King's site.

(v)   The conclusion of the Review Group is that in moving from the three current Centres to one, the unit that should close first is King's. The feasibility of this was demonstrated recently when the Guy's and St.Thomas' Units absorbed the radiotherapy workload of King's for an 18 month period whilst its Linac machine was being replaced. An additional linac is being installed at St. Thomas' and spare bunkers exist for further machines on both the Guy's and St. Thomas' site. (Some additional shielding may be needed). In view of this additional capacity, the Review recommends the early concentration from April 1994 of radiotherapy services on the Guy's and St.Thomas' sites.

(vi)   The Review Group was impressed by the commitment to create a Specialist Centre on one site expressed by both senior management and senior clinicians representing the newly combined Guy's and St. Thomas' Trust. This final move will create an exceptionally strong Cancer Centre for South East London.

(vii)   Although there are factors favouring the choice of either the St. Thomas'
or Guy's site for the South East London Cancer Centre; and these are
fairly evenly balanced, the Review Group concluded that taking into
account all of the information available, the Guy's site would be the
preferred option. The deciding factors include the Group's perception of
there being more available space on the Guy's site once the new
development is completed, the strength of the hospital's surgical and
medical oncology department, and the extent of investment, and the
track record in cancer research and development. It was considered that
the cancer research at St. Thomas' could be transferred to the Guy's site
to the long term benefit of both. However, all these issues will be minor
factors in the overall assessment of the two sites and the Review Group
would be perfectly content for either to be chosen, so long as the
particular strengths of both are consolidated. (A more detailed capital
appraisal is to be undertaken by the Trust).

(viii)   The impact of the excellent new facilities at Maidstone, opened in April
1993, in reducing the number of patients from Kent coming to the South
East London Centre is at present uncertain. However, it is anticipated
that the Maidstone Unit could well be economically expanded beyond its
design capacity and attract patients from nearer to London, eg. Bromley
which currently accounts for some 16% of SELRC's workload.

(ix)   The Review Group would envisage the strong Haematology Department
remaining at King's (see Haematology-oncology services in Section 6.8 of
the report). The Group does not believe that the removal of the small
radiotherapy service will undermine other specialist services provided on
site or its overall financial stability. (Cancer services represent less than
3% of its income). King's should retain a strong clinical and medical
oncology presence by a substantial outreach services from
Guy's/St.Thomas' Centre, as also proposed for St. George's and St.
Mary's Hospitals. This could well include joint appointments.

(x)   The proposed South East London Cancer Centre, on a single site, should
also include the only Academic Department of Palliative Care in England,
now at St. Thomas', which will continue to set standards and promote
improved care for the South East generally.

(xi)   The proposed South East London Cancer Centre could serve a population
of some 1.25M and so have the range of facilities envisaged for a unit
treating 4,000 new clinical/medical oncology patients per annum. The
level of capital investment needed to create the expanded Centre on the
Guy's site is estimated to be of the order of £10M.

(xii)   We believe that a single major oncology centre at either Guy's or St.
Thomas' would enable the available stills and facilities at all three sites to
enter a new phase of coordinated improvement in patient care and cancer
research.

7.5   THE SOUTH WEST AND WESTERN QUADRANT OF LONDON

7.5.1 Special factors in West London

Three different models of specialist cancer centres

In West London the key characteristics of the three main centres - Charing Cross Hospital, The Royal Marsden Hospital and The Hammersmith Hospital, differ significantly.

The Royal Marsden Hospital is a prime example of a single specialty institution, which has a substantial specialist medical training role and has traditionally been a major research centre.

Charing Cross hospital is an example of the predominant model in London, namely the multi-disciplinary undergraduate teaching hospital with specialist services.

The Hammersmith Hospital is the only example in the U.K. of a multi-specialty postgraduate teaching hospital, which also has research and development as a prime objective.

The smallest centre in London, with only two ortho-voltage radiotherapy machines, is at St. Mary's. This Unit accepts that it will not continue to have a radiotherapy department, and the Review proposes St. Mary's should become strongly linked to one of the other West London Units.

Particular Complexity

This is the most complex quadrant in which to recommend tenable proposals to translate the current arrangements for a future pattern that combines the many strengths in service, teaching and research that already exist.

One complicating and unique factor is that two of the units in close proximity in this quadrant are at present Special Health Authorities (the Royal Marsden and the Hammersmith). Nevertheless, changes in patient flows that are already gaining strength make it essential that reorganisation and consolidation should take place, and without delay.

Another factor is the likely reduction of patient flows to West London from the Oxford Region (see 7.4.3).

7.5.2 Profile of the services provided

WEST LONDON	CXH	H'SMITH	RM(F)	TOTAL
Total New Clinical Oncology Cases	3,000	1,850	~	4,850
Total RT Courses	3,715	1,853	2,100	7,668
Total RT Machines +	6 (6)	3 (4)	3 (5)	12 (15)
Total Chemotherapy Doses	22,000	11,600	13,000	46,600
Average Available Onc.Beds	69	25	111*	205
Total Bed Days	27,537	8,906	33,891**	70,334
# Income RT	£3.670M	£1.377M		
Chemotherapy	£2.254M	£3.069M	£23M**	
Haematology & Other	£3.117M	£3.681M		
% of the whole hospital revenue income represented by the above (% of whole hospital's capital charges).	5.8% (4.9%)	10.6% (9.7%)	100% (100%)	
Consultant Clinical & Medical Oncology Staff (WTE) ****	9.5	5.9	4.8	20.2
Senior Registrars/Registrars	11.0	5.5	10.0	26.5

~   The figures given to us by the Royal Marsden of 6,346 includes a quite different case-mix from any other unit in London with a high percentage of non-malignant diagnoses and surgical cases. This is analyzed separately below (   ).

+   Linear accelerators, cobalt machines and deep x-ray machines have been used as a proxy for the range of equipment available in 1992/93. Those in brackets show the extra ones commissioned since last year.

\#   Excluding capital charges.

*   This includes surgical beds and designated rehab. beds. Total beds on site 180. Some beds are closed.

**   £43M includes Sutton and Fulham Road sites. The Royal Marsden has not been able to give a complete breakdown between sites. As 53% of staff work at the Fulham Road Branch the revenue costs of the Fulham Road Branch are crudely estimated to be of the order of £23M. This indicates the high overhead costs of a small hospital on two sites, and high staff costs.

7.5.3 The units serve a dispersed population

Overall, the hospitals in this quadrant serve a more dispersed population with a less well defined core catchment than the Centres in the other three quadrants. This is particularly the case for The Royal Marsden Hospital. The prospects, confirmed by Health Authority representatives, is that these referral patterns will change as other Centres develop stronger links with their local DGHs. The future caseload in this sector is therefore more likely than the others to decline. Thus the flows to Charing Cross from Kent, based on an association with the former Westminster Unit are already declining; the new unit at Reading is likely to become the major Unit serving the East Berkshire district of the Oxford Region instead of the Hammersmith, and the flows from Surrey to the Royal Marsden, Fulham Road, are likely to be met increasingly by the Sutton branch, as it expands its size and range of services, and to some extent by Guildford when the new Centre, (now under construction) opens in 1995.

7.5.4 Referral Patterns

Charing Cross	Hammersmith	Royal Marsden* (Total for both sites).
660 (RTR)	555 (Ealing)	1420 (M & S)
600 (H & S)	370 (Berkshire)	708 (Mid Surrey)
450 (Croydon)	166 (Brent)	568 (Riverside)
300 (K & E)	93 (Harrow)	565 (K & E)
270 (Ealing)	74 (Hammersmith)	510 (RTR)
720 (Other)	592 (Other)	8020 (Others)
3000	1850	11,791

*   Of the total of 11,791 new patients, in 1991/92 the split between the two branches was 6,346 Fulham Road and 5,445 at Sutton. Of the total 10,680 were adults, with all the children being treated at Sutton.

The top referring districts shown provide just over a third of the total number of in-patients, almost a further 20% are provided by a further five districts and these constitute some 3,000 of the 8,020 others, the remaining 5,000 plus cases come from some 130 other districts.

7.5.5 Surplus capacity

All three Centres in West London have had, or are having, significant additional capacity created. (The number of Linacs is being increased overall by nearly 30%. There is scope for the current and future workload to be accommodated on only two or possibly only one site.

7.5.6 Strategic uncertainty

The Review Team does not believe it is practical at present to propose a single Centre for this part of London, given a number of uncertainties.

These include:-

- The importance which the SHA R & D Reviews will have for the future support of research and its added service costs in the quadrant. This will have fundamental implication for the Royal Marsden and Hammersmith Hospitals.

- The need for time to redefine the future of the unique postgraduate role of this part of London, in medical and non-medical training.

- The consequences of bringing the SHAs into the health care market.

- Alterations in referral pattern to the developing Centres at Reading and Guildford.

- Decisions on the future of the Charing Cross site and of the hospital's final case-mix if it remains open.

- The future range of services to be located at the Hammersmith.

- Possible changes in the referral pattern of acute cancer services in North West Outer London and their effect for the three centres.

Our belief is that, despite these uncertainties, the projected workload, at least in the short term, for one Centre in this part of London, would be above that envisaged for other units in the South East, and that it is safer to maintain two Centres at least for the time being.

7.5.7 Postgraduate education and research

These are important across the whole of London, but are dealt with here because of their special profile in this quadrant.

The advice received from all three Centres, and other Specialist Centres, is of the growing importance in postgraduate training of a multi-disciplinary (integrated care) approach to cancer care, i.e. oncology/radiotherapy and specialised surgery, as well as palliative care with their necessary supporting services, delivered by a team consisting of appropriate health care professionals. Both Charing Cross and (to almost as great an extent) the Hammersmith are well placed to provide this at present. The Royal Marsden Hospital is relatively weak in that although it has good new operating facilities at Fulham, most of its surgeons spend more of their time at other London hospitals than at the Marsden. At Sutton, there is only one theatre, used on a part time basis. The Royal Marsden has however for some years been seeking to remedy this aspect of its services. It plans to make further progress through closer links with the new Chelsea/Westminster Hospital, but still will not be able to achieve the same range or depth of specialised support at consultant and junior doctor level, (physically present rather than 'visiting' the site) as the other two hospitals. The Chelsea Westminster Hospital already has developed substantial visiting oncology services from Charing Cross Hospital.

The advice received on the future organisation of cancer research suggests that basic research will become more complex, and rely more on expensive equipment and specialised technical staff. Much of this research is likely to involve techniques applicable beyond the cancer field. Clinical research is also heavily dependent on a sufficiently high throughput of patients. This is currently a limitation for both the Hammersmith and Royal Marsden at Fulham, more than for the Charing Cross unit. It is more fully discussed in section 5.6.

AN ASSESSMENT OF THE THREE UNITS

7.5.8 Charing Cross Hospital

Access

(i)   Charing Cross, like the other two sites in this quadrant has a tube station within a 5-10 minute walk; it and the Royal Marsden, Fulham, are better served by bus routes than the Hammersmith. Like the Hammersmith, it has better road access for the West London population than the Royal Marsden (Fulham Road). Charing Cross has appreciably more on site car parking than the Hammersmith, which has more than the Royal Marsden (Fulham Road). Overall we consider that it has the best access of the three sites.

Facilities

(ii)   The newly built Radiotherapy Department at Charing Cross provides an excellent model in terms of the quality and layout of facilities for a large centre. It avoids an intimidating or impersonal atmosphere, and has clearly been well planned to minimise the tension felt by patients attending for cancer treatment. It is also capable of easy extension. The ward facilities are in an adjacent modern block with which communications are good. The ward layout provides good standards of privacy for patients with the adjacent for research labs, this facilitate close integration of clinical and research work.

(iii) A relatively well developed level of tumour site specialisation is already established amongst the 10 oncologists. It has the second largest medical oncology service in London after the Royal Marsden (Sutton). The chemotherapy area is larger and better laid out than the average seen, supporting a substantial medical oncology service. It could be brought closer to the main department in a new location, providing double the treatment space/stations. The unit provides a supra-regional service for choriocarcinoma. The haematology service is small with little acute leukaemia work being carried out.

Service Organisation

(iv) The unit has relatively well developed links with some district general hospitals compared with other centres in West London.

(v) At present, and subject to changes which may follow the other specialty reviews the unit has a strong multi specialty basis for treating cancer approaching that of the Royal London Hospital. Taking account of the recent opening of the Chelsea Westminster Hospital, Charing Cross has some 80 medical beds and 45 for care of the elderly, 26 renal beds and 100 surgical beds, leaving aside those in Regional specialties. This scale and range of specialty provision would provide an effective level of support for a major cancer centre on the Charing Cross Site and leaves a substantial margin for 'downsizing' before the range of this 'infrastructure' would become an issue. We believe some gynaecology beds would need to be located on site in future if the unit is to function fully as a major Cancer Centre.

(vi) The impact of the possible contraction of the A & E service would require further assessment, although its presence is not directly required for a Specialist Cancer Centre.

(vii) The presence of the West London Breast Screening Unit has led to the development of a well organised multi-disciplinary breast cancer service. There is also surgical sub-specialisation in gastrointestinal and urological cancer. Supra district specialties include ophthalmology, oral surgery and ENT which are committed to contributing to cancer treatment. At regional specialty level, the plastic surgery department is a particularly strong one and is involved in the complex treatment of major cancers requiring restorative surgery. Similarly the presence of neuro-sciences is important for the effective treatment of brain and spinal cord tumours. There is therefore a very broad base of services relevant to cancer treatment.

Research

(viii) The research strategy of the hospital is based on three major interests, namely neurosciences, vascular biology, and cell and molecular science of cancer. The breast cancer research unit is one of the largest in London. Both the ICRF and the CRC have a significant presence on site. The centre is well set up for cancer research both at the clinical level, through the close proximity of ward, and adjacent laboratories described above, but also through the site having a large amount of separate laboratory space. It was reported as having the largest animal house of any teaching hospital in London. The hospital is two tube stops from the Imperial College, with which it anticipates developing increasingly strong links both in basic research, and to provide undergraduate experience, particularly in a range of regional specialties. We believe that it should improve its research links with the RPMS/Hammersmith, and at basic service level, also, with Imperial College and the Institute of Cancer Research.

7.5.9 Hammersmith Hospital

Access

(i) The Unit has a tube station within 5-10 minutes walk, is less well served by bus routes, but has more car parking than the Royal Marsden (Fulham), but less than Charing Cross.

Facilities

(ii) The Unit is currently the smallest of the three with 1,850 new clinical/ medical oncology patients per annum. The facilities for cancer patients are currently of only average quality with the Radiotherapy Department being cramped and separate from other elements of the service which are also quite dispersed. Chemotherapy day facilities have been modernised and expanded in the last year and also provide a base for the Macmillan Nursing Team.

(iii) The new £5M Hammer Cancer Centre will transform the quality of most of the unit providing excellent facilities including wards, outpatients and a major new element of the Radiotherapy Department. Although the Unit had not planned to expand its workload following the new facilities opening in 1995, nevertheless on our capacity planning model the new development could provide for a modest increase with its existing equipment so that a little over 2,100 new patients could be treated per annum. Through a relatively modest further capital investment in the region of £2M with an extra simulator and Linac, an additional 700 or so new cases could be treated per annum. Expansion beyond the 2,800 new cases level would be however expensive and difficult to achieve, because of site constraints.

Service Organisation

(iv)   The Unit has developed in the last two years a stronger presence in a small number of DGHs in West London. However, the current geographical area it serves is not as well defined as would be needed to secure a workload approaching the minimum size necessary for high quality cancer services to be provided in the future. (23 districts refer less than ten in-patients p.a.; only three districts refer over 100 in-patients p.a.).

(v)   The Hospital has a range of exceptionally wide and high quality pathology services which could support an expanded cancer service to good effect.

(vi)   The surgical component of the cancer service does not cover all the main tumour types with the level of surgical sub-specialisation found in some other units. An enlarged unit would need a higher level of on site surgical commitment and sub-specialisation which would require a review of the current pattern of split appointments. There is a need particularly to reinforce colo-rectal cancer surgery. (The findings of the CEPOD reports, combined with advice to the Review Group from the Royal College of Surgeons, indicate that the appointment of surgeons to two hospitals both with emergency surgery commitments should not take place. Wherever possible surgeons should operate at a single site only).

(vii)   The clinical and medical oncologists have tumour specific interests although the small size of the department means this is less developed than in some other larger clinical oncology groups elsewhere in London.

(viii)   The Unit provides a number of particular services having the only cyclotron in London and also the MRC funded PET (positron emission tomography) programme. There is a strong haematology unit which works effectively with the rest of the cancer services provided on site.

Research

(ix)   The very substantial research commitment on the site involves the RPMS, ICRF, MRC, CRC and the Leukaemia Research Fund.

(x)   The RPMS has a proven record of good, relevant research. Its current programme received a high rating in the UFC selectivity exercise, and it is understood that the SHA research review is concluding similarly. The MRC has just established an important unit at Hammersmith, to carry out research in fields related to cancer. The ICRF also supports substantial research at the Hammersmith with four separate groups which together receive around £11M of the £55M total budget of the Fund. This unit works closely with the Fund's basic science laboratories in Lincoln's Inn Fields.

(xi)   The importance of the cancer research at RPMS is not only in cancer itself, but also in its close relevance to the medical research in other fields, to which it is complementary. Taken as a whole, it would we believe be very difficult and expensive to relocate it all to another site.

(xii)   We believe that links should nevertheless be strengthened between the RPMS/Hammersmith and Charing Cross, as well as with Imperial College so that both basic and clinical medical and especially cancer research in this quarter of London continues to have a sound base, using the principles described in section 5.3 for the relationships that are important for effective research.

7.5.10   The Royal Marsden (Fulham Road)

<u>Access</u>

(i)   The restricted site of 2.5 acres lies in a densely built up area, with little car parking for patients. It is well served by bus routes, a tube station is 5-10 minutes walk away, with Paddington and Victoria stations being the nearest main line termini.

<u>Facilities</u>

(ii)   The site has been intensively developed, both by new additions and extensive modernisation of the original ward blocks, although this has not been on the same scale as the neighbouring Royal Brompton Hospital. Nevertheless well in excess of £20M has been invested in the last five years, resulting in a suite of four new theatres with protected rooms for gynaecological radiotherapy treatments, two Linacs, and a major ward and catering development have recently been opened, all being of an excellent standard. As a consequence the unit currently has 50% spare theatre capacity (excluding the selectron suite, where 8 of the 10 sessions are booked), and has 30% spare capacity, given the increased number of Linacs that now exist. There are two simulator and planning systems, and CT is available, but not MRI.

(iii)   The Hospital has 180 beds, including 19 designated for hostel use, 13 for palliative care, 6 high dependency unit and 30 beds are currently not in use.

(iv)   The Radiotherapy Department falls into the common pattern we observed of a basement location, so that although various improvements had been achieved, the inherent limitations in its layout remain. The Department does not compare with the quality of facilities or the patient focused design of the Charing Cross Unit, or of that now under construction at the Hammersmith Hospital.

(v)   As in many units visited, the Chemotherapy service had good quality treatment facilities, but poorly laid out cytotoxic drug preparation areas. The service is approximately the same size as that of Hammersmith Hospital, but a little over half the size of that provided by Charing Cross. Much of the intensive chemotherapy for adults and all of that for children is carried out at Sutton.

Service Organisation - Staffing Profile

(vi)   The staffing profile is different in a number of significant respects from that seen elsewhere, and so we have examined it in some detail. From the information provided, it has not been possible to separate as clearly as we would have liked, the staffing arrangements for the two sites.

-       The complement of 70 consultant staff for the 2 sites contains a higher proportion than elsewhere of shared appointments. In many cases the consultant's main base is another hospital. Some (especially surgeons) even work at more than two. Given the exceptionally large group of oncologists, a high level of tumour sub-specialisation has been achieved which has assisted not just service quality, but also the organisation of research.

        The pattern of largely part time surgeons with an interest in oncology but based primarily at other hospitals, has been recognised as a problem for the unit which they have been addressing for some years. With the appointment very recently of a new Research Director (the Professor of Surgery) the hospital aims to address this to resolve it as a problem.

-       The presence of 33 junior medical training posts across the two sites is substantially higher than any other Centre in London, or indeed the rest of the country. (It is over a third of London's total of 80 such posts). It should be remembered that Registrars, and especially Senior Registrars, usually make a significant contribution to service (unless wholly engaged in non-clinical research).

-       The two sites have some 335 whole time equivalent nurses excluding haemato-oncology and paediatric oncology, which again is substantially higher than any other unit. This is principally associated with the large number of beds which the unit has and the fact that surgical bed use for many non malignant conditions is included, unlike other Centres.

-       The predominant role of the unit in specialist nurse training programmes also contributes to the high number of nurses, but to a lesser extent than the ward staffing component.

-      The Radiographer and Physics staffing numbers are higher than
       might be expected for the workload by comparison with other
       units, but there is a strong radiotherapy physics research unit at
       Sutton.

Clinical Units

(vii)   There are 16 clinical units, most of which are not duplicated on each site.
        The result is that patients are referred in both directions, and may need to
        undergo aspects of their care, on occasions, at both hospitals.

(viii) Four of the I6 clinical units are entirely on the Fulham Road site; those for
        gynaecology, head and neck cancer, skin and melanoma, and soft tissue
        sarcoma. (Seven specialty groups are at Sutton - paediatric, GI tract,
        myeloma, lung, clinical pharmacology, neuro-oncology and thyroid
        cancer). There is, however, almost no surgery in connection with these
        cancers at Sutton. Both sites provide a service for breast cancer and
        blood related malignancies, palliative care and psychological support,
        urology and testicular cancer. These complexities have made it
        necessary for the Review Group to analyze the patient statistics in some
        detail to obtain a clearer picture. In doing so we have used our own
        collected data, and also some submitted with the Royal Marsden's
        response to the Director of Research and Development for the research
        SHA review. (Appendix 10.7)

The Review Group's own analysis of the Workload

(ix)   Of the 10,680 new adult patients registered in 1991/92 and analyzed in
        the table in Appendix 10.6, 5,976 had a malignant diagnosis and the
        remaining 4,704, therefore, had benign conditions. We have presumed
        that this latter figure includes the 2,000 women with an increased risk of
        developing breast cancer, who are taking part in a study comparing
        tamoxifen treatment against a placebo. In most of the tumour sites
        listed, however, the unit identifies a quite substantial number of non
        malignant cases - far more than would be seen at other cancer centres.
        Of the 5,976 patients with a malignant diagnosis many (G.I. tract, skin,
        urology) would not, however, have been registered by other oncology
        centres since they would have been treated entirely by surgery alone.
        Nor would the internal referrals for palliative and psychological medicine
        (549) have been separately counted as new malignant cases. It is not
        clear how many of the patients registered were only seen for a second
        opinion and not thereafter treated at the Royal Marsden.

(x)   Taking these figures, and relating them to the current balance of service
        provision at the two branches (60% of the work is carried out at Sutton,
        we were told) we believe that the Fulham Road branch is currently
        treating some 1,500 to 2,000 new non surgical cancer patients per year.
        In other centres, for example Mount Vernon, we have found that there is

an approximate numerical equivalence between the number of new oncology cases registered and the total number of new radiotherapy courses of treatment administered. This would give a similar figure of around 2,000 patients for Fulham Road, or rather less if there are a larger than usual number of patients who only come to the Royal Marsden for a second opinion, not treatment. The more recent information supplied by the hospital indicates 2,100 radiotherapy courses in 1991/92 which confirms the level of work we have deduced is reasonably accurate.

(xi)   These workload figures show an increase from the figure of 1,490 new oncology cases treated at its Fulham Road branch that the Royal Marsden gave as their radiotherapy and oncology workload to the Royal College of Radiologists for its 1990 survey.

(xii)   We believe that these figures taken together are a reasonable estimate of the radiotherapy and medical oncology workload at Fulham Road, which is considerably below the minimum size we believe is appropriate for a cancer centre in an urban area.

(xiii)   Some 10% of the overall workload involves the treatment of less common and rare tumours. This work is, however, predominantly carried out at the Sutton branch and will be covered below.

(xiv)   There is a high level of inpatient admission to both branches of the Royal Marsden Hospital, with some 13,370 inpatient episodes across the two sites in 1991/92. Some 18% of the beds are filled by private and overseas patients, although the total of patients seen in these groups is only 12% of the whole. This latter figure is only a little higher than the number in some other London units.

(xv)   75% of the chemotherapy treatments administered were at the Sutton branch, as were all the 140 bone marrow transplants carried out in 1991/92.

(xvi)   Considering the workload of the hospital as a whole, it is clear that it has a fundamental difference from that of other cancer centres. Much of the work being carried out at Fulham Road would be carried out in the general and especially surgical services of multi-specialty hospitals, as well as in local acute units. There does not seem any overriding reason why this relatively general, although cancer related, work could not be achieved just as satisfactorily by patients following the normal pattern of care that is available to them in other places, and which we are proposing for the other major cancer centres in and near London, provided that it is of the quality standards that we recommend.

(xvii) Whilst historically there may have been reasons for an unusual balance of cases being referred to the Royal Marsden, nowadays the quality of surgical and the specialist cancer care in local acute hospitals makes this unnecessary. Given the trend to greater surgical specialisation in DGHs and the limitations of the Royal Marsden's surgical capacity, we have concluded that much of its Fulham Road work will over time be dealt with elsewhere.

Role in Treating Less Common Cancers

(xviii) The Royal Marsden Hospitals have had a particular interest in treating less common and rare cancers.

(xix) Between the two branches, some 1,100 new cancer cases are seen per annum in these categories, which represents just over l0% of the total workload of the two sites. They include children's cancer, soft tissue sarcomas and other rare cancers. They are predominantly treated at the Sutton branch. There are however, no supra-Regional cancer services based at the Royal Marsden, although three such services are based at other London cancer centres.

Referral Patterns

(xx) Ten District Health Authorities provide 50% of the in-patients, these are predominantly from the South West Thames Region, but a number also come from North West Thames. A further 130 districts each refer less than 2% of the total workload of the unit. The service provided for these remote districts is predominantly in the treatment of common rather than rare cancers, and usually derives from long established referral patterns. In the future, cost and access is likely to result in many of these patients being referred locally, with the improved cancer treatment centres now developing outside London.

(xxi) The Royal Marsden Hospital, Fulham Road, was the only Centre visited in the South East where consultants had not established any outreach clinics where their oncology specialists hold sessions in local District General Hospitals.

Research & Development

(xxii) We have not sought to duplicate the separate review of the R & D performance of the SHAs, but have limited our views to the impact which research has on the service provided by hospital and the other cancer services in London. The Royal Marsden Hospital has estimated that its two sites need some 5,600 new cases of malignant disease annually to support its research (this corresponds closely to the current level of referrals for its research programme). The unit acknowledges however that the number of patients needed to support the hospital as an NHS provider would be significantly higher than this, having regard to the relatively low number of specialist non-surgical treatments to which this gives rise, on both sites.

(xxiii) The association of the Royal Marsden Hospital with the Institute of Cancer Research is well known. It has led to many productive co-developments, but there are also areas where research is pursued separately in the hospital or the Institute settings.

(xxiv) This review has not been able to consider in any depth the research potential of the Royal Marsden hospital which derives from its close association with the ICR. That, we felt, was work to which the SHA review of research and development would contribute. We have however tried to form a view, from discussions with leaders in laboratory and clinical cancer research on the need for a close geographical link between the Fulham Road hospital, and the adjacent Institute. We have concluded from this that whilst this juxta position does have advantages in allowing useful discussions between clinical and research staff, there are no other particular features which make this on-site link essential to support future relevant research. We believe that basic cancer science links should be strengthened between the Royal Marsden at Sutton and the ICR and Imperial College, and that in such a strengthening the future outlook for research will be if anything better than it has been in the past. Much of the Institute's good current research - in physics and in drug development for instance - is already based at Sutton. Our general note and recommendations for cancer research in section 5.6 apply as much to the Royal Marsden as elsewhere, we believe.

Training and Education

(xxv) The presence of 28 registrar and senior registrar posts reflects the substantial postgraduate medical training role carried out for many years by the unit. This will undergo significant change as the final objectives of JPAC are achieved, by which the total registrar numbers in the U.K. are to be reduced by some 50%. There will in consequence be approved training posts available in many other Cancer Centres in the country. JPAC considers that the planned numbers of trainees should still be sufficient to fill the consultant expansion anticipated in 'Achieving a Balance'. This number may well not meet the needs if the Government implement the Calman Report.

(xxvi) The first postgraduate nursing courses started in 1960 with the unit being the first in the U.K. to offer specialist post-basic courses in 1975. These have now developed to cover a range of disciplines, e.g. with intravenous training, stoma care nurses and breast cancer nurse specialists. The first rehabilitation department, including a lymphodema therapy service, was introduced in 1988, and the first academic nurse research unit was created in 1990.

(xxvii) The record of training in nursing and allied professions has been outstanding, with 80% of specialist oncology nurses having trained at the Marsden. Now however, this training is becoming available elsewhere, so that it should not be necessary for staff to travel to London for this to the same extent.

7.5.11 Future plans of the Royal Marsden Hospitals

<u>Chelsea Health Sciences Centre Concept</u>

(i)   The plan of the Royal Marsden Hospital is to remain operating on two sites and strengthen its linkages with other local Institutions, principally through the Chelsea Health Sciences Centre (CHSC) concept proposed by the Hospital as part of its response to the Tomlinson Report. (This report had recommended the unit's transfer to the Charing Cross Site). The CHSC proposal involves the Royal Brompton, Chelsea Westminster and the Royal Marsden Hospitals linking together with Imperial College, thereby sharing clinical expertise, some support services and most importantly co-ordinating research, while retaining their separate Institutional identities.

(ii)   From the perspective of the best possible organisation of cancer services for West London we believe that the CHSC concept only offers limited advantages. Neither the Brompton, nor Chelsea Westminster Hospitals have the relevant range of specialties to overcome the current limitations of the Royal Marsden, e.g. they also lack specialties such as neuro-sciences, plastic surgery, ENT and oral surgery. Furthermore the dispersed pattern of services spread over several sites in the CHSC arrangement would not in our view provide an integrated service in the same way as locating cancer services on a multi-specialty site.

(iii)   The CHSC would fail to draw together the nearby existing research grouping, with significant overlapping interests, at Charing Cross and the Hammersmith with those of the Royal Marsden, Fulham Road.

(iv)   The conclusion of the Review is that, as currently proposed, the CHSC proposal would not resolve the underlying problems which it is believed the Royal Marsden Hospital faces. Nevertheless the Review Group does believe that there is great advantage in a wider group of Institutions (including Hammersmith and Charing Cross) within West London forming a closer relationship with Imperial College, as well as its other important links with the Institute of Cancer Research. This larger collaborative grouping would provide a better basis for undergraduate and postgraduate medical education, as well as more powerful research units than the current fragmented arrangements, or the partial link-up represented by the CHSC proposal.

(v)   The Royal Marsden has emphasised the lack of effective collaborative cancer research programmes in London at present. We believe that this will be best addressed, as we recommend, by:-

- Linking larger cancer centres to a strong university base.

- Increasing cancer centres to a critical mass of patients and broadly based research skills.

- In West London, a better synergy between Imperial College and all of the existing and future cancer centre(s).

- In Surrey, strengthening research links between the Royal Marsden and St. George's.

A Comprehensive Cancer Centre

(vi)   The Royal Marsden, in their submission to the Tomlinson Inquiry, and also to the Review Group, have emphasised their wish to be regarded as a Comprehensive Cancer Centre.

(vii)   The International Union against Cancer (UICC) has proposed two distinct types of Specialist Cancer Centre, namely:-

- Cancer Centres designated within a main general hospital, which provides screening, general surgery, medical oncology and radiotherapy services for common cancers, supported by sophisticated diagnostic facilities for a local catchment population of around a million people.

- Comprehensive Cancer Centres - independent facilities that integrate diagnosis, patient care, research and education. Each would fulfil the role of a Cancer Centre, together with a specialised function in the treatment of rare disease, genetic screening, rehabilitation, palliative care, and an extensive research programme in a significant commitment to education and training of the clinical professions.

(viii)   The assessment of the Review Group is that the Royal Marsden Hospital in its current form is not well placed to achieve this objective, because:-

- The future pattern of a smaller number of larger Centres in London, each with good research links, across a range of specialties, including cancer, means that a Comprehensive Cancer Centre would be a difficult concept to introduce in London in terms of research organisation, nor is it supported by a wide selection of leaders in cancer research whom we have consulted.

- A number of other Centres have already achieved DoH recognition in providing supra-Regional services - Charing Cross, the Middlesex and St. Bartholomew's in London. Others already provide a valued and established service for particular cancers of less rare types.

- The Fulham Road Branch of the Royal Marsden Hospital does not at present provide a comprehensive local service to a population approaching a million people, on which the more specialist work would need to be based.

- Most of the treatment of rarer cancers is concentrated at the Sutton, rather than Fulham Road branch.

- The pattern of innovation in cancer care is already following a dispersed pattern, and restructuring this is seen as impractical, as well as inappropriate in our view.

- The pattern of a large number of surgeons with an interest in cancer from many difficult hospitals each working a few sessions at the Royal Marsden is not one that is supported by the surgical specialist associations of the Royal College of Surgeons. We believe that it is not well placed to promote advances in multi-modality care involving complex surgery.

(ix)   Other strategic issues which need to be addressed concerning the plans of the Royal Marsden Hospital, are its intention to set up a Health Evaluation Unit with the Royal Brompton Hospital, that it become the National Cancer Trials Centre, the proposal to establish a £15M 'Breakthrough Unit' for Breast Cancer Treatment, and the proposal that non-medical education and training should be based in the Institute of Cancer Research. In our view none of these is necessarily require retention of the Fulham Road site.

7.5.12 Our assessment of the possibilities of service expansion at Fulham Road

The Royal Marsden's Proposal

(i)   With the two additional Linacs installed at the Royal Marsden, Fulham Road, the unit could expand on that site from treating 2,100 up to 3,600 new courses per annum. If a 6th Linac were to be installed in a vacant bunker, then the unit indicates a further 900 cases could be accommodated to give the potential capacity of 4,500 courses. The new theatre development could also absorb this, more than doubling of the current workload. There is more limited scope to expand outpatient and inpatient facilities.

Service Organisation Problems

(ii)   The obstacles to the Royal Marsden, Fulham, achieving this doubling of its current workload are in our view substantial:-

- The location of the Royal Marsden, Fulham Road is not as readily accessible to serve a larger population in West London as are the

-89-

Hammersmith and Charing Cross Hospitals, in relation to the M4 and M40 or the tube and rail routes coming from West London.

- The absence of any outreach clinics by oncology specialists based at Fulham Road to DGHs in West London, makes it unlikely that an increased level of referrals will occur. Indeed as other Centres strengthen their presence in local acute hospitals, referrals are likely to reduce. The CHSC concept might mean clinics are established at the Chelsea Westminster Hospital, although Charing Cross which is part of the same Trust already has a strong presence on the Chelsea Westminster site.

- Our concern for the Royal Marsden in this regard has been reinforced by Health Authority representatives, emphasising the importance they place on a strong oncology presence in local general hospitals as a way of introducing more 'seamless', patient focused care and to prevent 'unnecessary referrals'.

- The pattern of so much consultant medical and surgical care being given by, as the Marsden describes, 'part-time consultants working in undergraduate hospitals' is we regard a further problem in terms of continuity of care.

- We also believe the pattern of 'visiting consultants' is a contributory factor to the high number of beds, and hence ward costs, that is apparent compared with other London units.

- We believe that even if these physical constraints could be overcome, the site is already very intensively developed, and that this would leave no margin for future expansion.

- The hospital would remain a single specialty cancer centre.

Expansion on the Fulham Road site is unlikely to happen

(iii)   The conclusion of the Review Team is therefore that the Royal Marsden Hospital, Fulham Road, will have substantial difficulty in retaining the existing level of referrals. Furthermore, that the costs of the Royal Marsden service, on the evidence available, are likely to be significantly higher than those of other Centres, which will also inhibit the achievement of the expansion plans of the hospital.

7.5.13 Future Of The Royal Marsden (Sutton)

(i)   The Review Group's analysis of the situation of the Sutton Branch of the Royal Marsden hospital is much more optimistic, as the unit is the most convenient Specialist Centre for a sizeable population in South London and Surrey and, unlike the Fulham Road Branch, the unit has a number of outreach clinics in neighbouring local acute hospitals. It is an established main Centre for the treatment of some rarer cancers, as well as being a principal site for specialist treatment techniques, and specialist diagnostic services such as MR imaging and spectroscopy and nuclear medicine. The site being ten times larger than the Fulham Road one, also has the prospect of more effective utilisation and expansion.

(ii)   A more detailed examination of the Sutton Branch of the Royal Marsden Hospital is included in Section 8 of this report.

Drawbacks of split site working of The Royal Marsden Hospitals

(iii)   The split site working between the Fulham Road and Sutton branches (they are twelve miles apart) has in recent years led to each developing a different role, so that now neither provides a comprehensive service to the separate geographical areas that they naturally serve. The Review Team was concerned about the effect this has had in increasing the distance patients have to travel and on communication and continuity of care; (mirroring the drawbacks identified for the Guy's, King's and Thomas' situation in South East London). Much staff time is also wasted on travel between sites. The Review Team was re-assured that the Hospital felt this arrangement could be reversed.

(iv)   The split of work between the Fulham Road and Sutton branches also reflects a lack of close working with other institutions e.g. all lung cancer work is concentrated at Sutton, despite the Fulham Road branch being adjacent to the Royal Brompton Hospital, with a unique level of expertise in lung disease. Paediatric oncology services are not within the remit of this Review Group. Nevertheless it was noted that children's services are located at the Sutton branch where the availability of paediatric expertise is less than that available in central London e.g. from the Westminster Children's Hospital now located within the Chelsea/Westminster Hospital.

(v)   The NHS workload is approximately one third larger at the Sutton Branch. If a more complete service was offered, the Fulham Road workload would become even smaller,

(vi)   The view of the Group, is that research as well as services to patients must have been damaged by these split site working arrangements reducing the effective work time, and the opportunity for daily interchange of ideas.

An Opportunity For The Royal Marsden To Centralise On One Site

(vii)   The Fulham Road site is a restricted one, which does not have the capacity to absorb the Sutton branch, although as previously described some of the facilities could be used more intensively than is currently the case. Centralisation on the Fulham Road site would be contrary to the principle established by the Group of sustaining a network of Centres in outer London where large concentrations of population exist. If the Sutton Branch closed, this population would have to travel substantially further for their treatment. (Guildford, Chelsea, Guy's/St. Thomas', Maidstone or even for some in the south, Brighton)

(viii)   Centralising on the Sutton site appears a much better option.

- The site is some ten times larger than the Fulham Road one, which gives it the capacity to do a larger range and volume of work, although its surgical capacity is limited.

- There is no other specialist cancer centre in close proximity to the Unit, and it therefore has a large natural population to serve.

- It has a network of outreach clinics in DGHs, which also provide a more secure referral base. than the Fulham Road Branch.

- 75% of the Group's chemotherapy workload is carried out at Sutton. The Marsden reported that it currently has 25% of the national training programme for senior registrars in medical oncology. The Sutton site therefore has a major training role in this growing specialty.

- Most of the treatment of rare cancers is already centred at Sutton, as are specified treatment techniques.

- The additional space on the Sutton site, compared with the Fulham Road site, will provide the best guarantee that the important national training contribution to specialist nurse education and other disciplines is protected and developed in the future.

- There is already a large research presence including some of the better known units - for example, radiation physics and the drug development unit.

These issues will be covered further in our recommendations for out of London centres, in Section 8, below.

7.5.14 Possible re-location of the Fulham Road Branch to a multi-specialty site in London

(i)   The relative advantages have been examined of the Fulham Road branch of the Marsden moving to the Hammersmith or Charing Cross Sites. The Review Team has concluded that if such was to occur, Charing Cross would be the preferable location to secure for the Royal Marsden a future as a major force in delivering cancer services of high quality allied to a significant national research and teaching role. This is based on the following factors:-

- Charing Cross has a larger, more modern set of facilities, and more vacant good quality ward accommodation, than the Hammersmith.

- The Charing Cross site has available good quality space to accommodate the Royal Marsden's substantial research units.

- Charing Cross subject to the results of other specialty reviews, will have a wider range of specialties than the Hammersmith particularly those relevant to cancer services, e.g. plastic surgery, ENT and neuro-sciences.

- Charing Cross staff expressed a strong wish to become the major centre serving West London. Conversely the Hammersmith Hospital expressed reservations, given the overall site constraints, the more limited size of the existing cancer unit and the underlying commitment of the Institution to preserving a wider range of more moderately sized specialties for its prime postgraduate research and teaching role.

- The arrangements for expanding the Charing Cross Radiotherapy Department to a 5 or 6 Linac Centre are well defined and could be carried out at relatively low cost without compromising the high quality, patient focused service arrangements that have already been created.

(ii) However, although the Charing Cross has the capacity to absorb the patients now cared for at the Royal Marsden (Fulham) we have concluded this is a less desirable option than unifying the two branches of the Royal Marsden on its main (Sutton) site. Our principal reasons for this conclusion are:-

- We believe the interdependence of the two Branches of the Royal Marsden Hospital is complex at a number of levels in service, teaching and research terms. Splitting the Royal Marsden with part being absorbed into Charing Cross, would be more disruptive and perhaps in the end less successful than allowing the hospital itself to control its own relocation from Fulham Road to its Sutton site.

- While West London has more Specialist Cancer Centres and capacity than the current need, and more particularly the future likely referral patterns will sustain, the Royal Marsden, Sutton, is the only conveniently located Specialist Centre for a large area of South London and parts of Surrey. Building up the Royal Marsden by centralising its activities at Sutton will therefore offer the SHA greater security that the patient workload will be large enough to sustain the Hospital continuing to have a major teaching and research role.

- Unifying the two Branches of the Royal Marsden Hospital on the Sutton site, offers overall the opportunity for the Institution to be strengthened, rather than weakened by continuing to be split and part being absorbed into another institution (Charing Cross).

(iii)   The Review Group believes the limitations of a single-specialty setting of the Royal Marsden, Sutton Branch, is best addressed by developing a range of closer linkages with the St. George's Trust. This is considered further in section 8.

(iv)   The proposed arrangements for single site (Sutton) operation would not disadvantage Chelsea patients, since there is, and would remain, ample specialist capacity for their care at Charing Cross. Only a very few patients with rare conditions might need to travel to Sutton (as might others from elsewhere in London or further afield).

7.5.16 The Way Forward for the South West and West London Quadrant

(i)   For different reasons the Royal Marsden, Hammersmith and Charing Cross all have undoubted strengths but there are some uncertainties around each being a suitable base for a major centre in the future.

Charing Cross Hospital

(ii)   Subject to the hospital's range of specialties being confirmed, the Review has concluded that the Charing Cross Site provides the best of the three locations for the main Specialist Cancer Centre for West London. The principal reasons being:-

- It is the most accessible.

- It has the best quality facilities overall at present.

- It has a greater range and volume of related specialties that are important for cancer services in the future, than the other two centres.

- It has the available space to expand more economically than the other two sites in the context of a strong multi-specialty service being a pre-requisite.

- It has a large, good quality, on site research capacity.

- Its referral pattern seems the most secure of the three hospitals.

Hammersmith Hospital

(iii)   The Hammersmith Hospital, being marginally the smallest of the three units in West London, would superficially seem the obvious Centre to relocate to the Charing Cross Site, particularly as our analysis would suggest that it is unlikely to expand above the minimum size regarded as acceptable for a Specialist Centre in the future. The Review Group is aware that representatives of Hammersmith Hospital are examining the possibility of relocating to the Charing Cross site, compared with remaining at the Hammersmith Hospital.

(iv)   An ideal solution from the Review Group's point of view would be for an early agreement that the Hammersmith and Charing Cross Units would combine on the latter site, while preserving the research and general postgraduate medical role of the Hammersmith/RPMS. However our conclusion is that this complicated situation will take some considerable time to resolve, given the significance of the Hammersmith in the national research programme, which in our belief (but subject to the SHA research review) needs to be protected. Nevertheless given the small size of the cancer service unit, it has little scope for absorbing reductions in workload, without becoming uneconomic in service terms, and as a consequence, its future research potential being compromised.

(v)   The Review Group believes that the Hammersmith Hospital should expand the current size of its service somewhat by absorbing the **St. Mary's** non-surgical cancer services so that it can expand to near the minimum size we recommend. We believe that the importance of the research and general postgraduate medical role of the Hammersmith is of such significance that the drawbacks of its relatively small size are likely to be compensated to a substantial degree for the foreseeable future. This will depend amongst other things upon the outcome of the SHA research review and subsequent funding for service costs of research.

(vi)   Furthermore, the continued presence of the cancer unit on the Hammersmith site gives flexibility vis-a-vis the longer term pattern of services. If referrals in West London are sufficient, both Charing Cross and Hammersmith will be viable (accepting that support for the added service costs of research is forthcoming). If not, an amalgamation of the two units will need to be sought.

(vii) It is recommended that the Hammersmith Hospital's cancer services develop closer working links with the expanded Charing Cross Unit.

The Royal Marsden Hospitals

(viii) The Review Group recognises the strength of public support for the Royal Marsden Hospital, and so sees as one of its key objectives sustaining the best features of the hospital, so giving it a new impetus to make a major contribution to advances in the treatment of cancer in the future.

(ix)   The Review Group has concluded that the best way forward is for Marsden to concentrate its future service and clinical research on an expanded Sutton Branch, where an exceptionally strong Centre could thereby be established.

(x)   To achieve this, the Review Group recommends that the management of the Royal Marsden Hospitals should be joined with the St. George's Trust, and a carefully planned process of change set in motion. (Section 8 of the report describes the reasons for the proposed joining of St. George's and the Royal Marsden Sutton Branch).

(xi)   The consequential reorganisation of research activities, particularly the Institute for Cancer Research, would need careful examination, based on the differing extent to which various research groups work need to work particularly closely with clinicians.

7.5.16 A Further Review

The Review Group believes that the North West Thames RHA and local Health Authorities, in conjunction with national research and teaching interests, should review within three years the roles being fulfilled by the two remaining specialist Cancer Centres in West London, namely the Hammersmith and the Charing Cross Units. By that time a number of issues will have been clarified.

-        The role of the Hammersmith is likely to have become more clearly defined following its entry into the internal market, and the impact of R & D funding support becoming apparent.

-        The North West Thames RHA in conjunction with the Oxford, and possibly North East Thames and East Anglia RHA's, and relevant local Health Authorities will have reached a decision on where patients living in the North of the Region should have specialist cancer services provided - whether by expansion of the Northampton Unit or by a new Centre in the north of the North West Thames Region.

-        The impact of the Oxford Region having a higher level of self sufficiency in Berkshire will also be clearer.

-        The patient flows that will arise from the new pattern of services developed between the North Middlesex and the Middlesex Centres will also be more clear.

7.5.17 Capital Implications

(i)   At the Hammersmith, the existing Radiotherapy Department would require some adaptations to bring it up to the standards of the new Hammer Cancer Centre as would some support service areas. The estimated costs would be no more than £500,000.

(ii)   At Charing Cross the chemotherapy area would need expanding, and an additional linac bunker provided again costing in total under £1M.

(iii)   The major cost but also largest capital receipt centres around the relocation of the Marsden from Fulham Road. The outpatient area at Sutton is not up to the standard of most of the rest of the hospital, the chemotherapy areas would probably also need expanding, however the main cost would be in relocating research units, if it is determined that these costs would fall to the NHS. Overall we have assumed a sum of £5M. The savings in dual site revenue costs, would we believe re-pay this in three years approximately, leaving aside the impact of any land sales.

7.6   THE NORTH LONDON QUADRANT

7.6.1 Access

The Royal Free Hospital and UCH/Middlesex Hospital are situated in this quadrant of inner London. They are within four miles of each other and they are linked by a tube route being six stops apart. Both have relatively small radiotherapy units but large oncology services. The close proximity of the North Middlesex and of St. Mary's Hospitals is also relevant to provision in this quadrant.

7.6.2 Profile of the service

NORTH LONDON	UCH/MIDDX	ROYAL FREE	TOTAL
Total New Clinical Oncology Cases	2,800	1,221	4,021
Total RT Courses	3,208	1,016	4,224
+ Total RT Machines	6 (6)	3 (4)	9 (10)
Total Chemotherapy Doses	Not available	7,600	------
*Total Onc.Bed Days	19,090	8,614	27,704
Average Available Onc.Beds	64	24	88
**Income RT	£6,299,000	£2,140,000	£8,439,000
Chemotherapy	£1,185,000	£764,000	£11,835,000
Haematology & Other	£5,465,000	£6,370,000	
% of the whole hospital revenue income represented by the above (% of whole hospital's capital charges)	9.4% (9.4%)	10.6% (7.9%)	
Consultant Clinical and Medical Oncology Staff (WTE)	4.9	3.1	8.0

+   Linear accelerators, cobalt and deep x-ray machines have been used as a proxy for the full range of equipment available (1992/3).
*   Includes medical and clinical oncology cases.
**   Exc. capital charges

Source: Returns from centres (1991/92 unless otherwise stated).

7.6.3 Main districts referring patients

The current referral patterns of the two hospitals and access for the populations served is very similar for the two sites. Both units draw mainly from the north and west with the Royal Free having a smaller flow of patients from the east. There is also an overlap with the present catchment area of the Hammersmith, Mount Vernon, and the North Middlesex. This has made it difficult for us to be definite about future purchasing patterns.

UCH/Middlesex	The Royal Free
521 (H & S) 462 (Bloomsbury & Islington) 258 (Parkside) 235 (Barnet) 134 (E & N.Herts) 1190 (Other)	348 (Barnet) 302 (Hampstead) 75 (Haringey) 72 (E & N.Herts) 70 (Bloomsbury & Islington) 354 (Other)
2800	1221

7.6.4 Common features

The Royal Free Hospital and the UCH/Middlesex Hospital share a number of other features:-

- Each has a large and well developed oncology service with a strong research record.

- Both have a particularly large haematology service (two of the four largest of the thirteen main centres in the capital).

- The two units share a Palliative Care Team which serves a population of 300,000 covering Islington, Hampstead and Bloomsbury.

- The two units also have particular expertise in treatment of tumours of the nervous system. There is good surgical and oncology site specialisation at both hospitals. Colo-rectal cancer is an established area of expertise of the Royal Free; This is likely to be complemented by a parallel interest at UCH/Middlesex Hospital, following the appointment there of a new Professor of Surgery, and the research group that has transferred with him.

7.6.5 A single centre for North Central London

(i)   The Royal Free Hospital's Radiotherapy Unit is well below the minimum size we have defined to provide a comprehensive, high quality service to the people in this part of London requiring specialist cancer services. Its catchment area would only increase sufficiently to change this if it took on the UCH/Middlesex patients, or in the event of closure of the North Middlesex which we do not recommend (see section 8). We cannot see that it will remain viable to retain radiotherapy or intensive medical oncology services on both the Royal Free and the Middlesex sites, even in the short to medium term.

(ii)   By combining the two large medical oncology units, a service would be created that would be one of the strongest in London and would have a particularly advanced research base, bringing together the high quality work taking place on both sites. The two units already carry out joint projects, have closely linked research programmes, and they already have an agreement to aim to create a single academic medical oncology department on one site.

(iii)   The combined unit would have considerable surgical sub-specialisation in oncology, particularly in breast and colo-rectal cancer, neuro-oncology, and in soft tissue and bone sarcomas. It could well also, bearing in mind existing links with the Hospital for Sick Children at Great Ormond Street, become the principal off-site support for that hospital's needs, for children.

7.6.6 Assessment of the two sites

(i)   In many respects the choice between the two sites is evenly balanced in terms of service accessibility to a larger population. Both sites have a number of advantages with regard to being the location of the new merged centre as set out below.

<u>General Issues</u>

(ii)   The Royal Free Hospital is the more spacious site. The building is only twenty years old and has a basic layout that is closer to the needs of the future eg. more spacious wards, and flexibility to provide patient focused services. The infrastructure of the hospital is more modern.

(iii)   The Royal Free Hospital is the main hospital for a larger 'natural catchment population' and is perhaps better guaranteed to have a reasonable range and volume of general acute services that are important to support a specialist cancer unit. Colo-rectal and breast surgery services are particularly strong at the Royal Free.

(iv)   The Royal Free Unit's income has remained stable since the introduction of the internal market, whereas the UCH/Middlesex Unit has suffered significant losses. As a consequence the latter has been going through a major rationalisation of its existing sites, which has now largely been completed. The prices of the Royal Free are amongst the lowest of the London Teaching Hospitals. Prices at UCH/Middlesex Unit are less disaggregated and so are difficult to compare, but appear higher overall.

(v)   The conclusion is that in terms of general issues relating to site suitability, financial stability and a reasonably well defined and balanced future pattern of services, the Royal Free might be the preferable site as compared with the UCH/Middlesex.

Cancer service issues

(vi)   In examining the cancer services specifically however the UCH/Middlesex centre is seen as having the following advantages:-

-     The Radiotherapy Centre is the larger of the two units and therefore closer to the proposed size for a future centre. It would be more economical to expand, although at both sites this would be more costly than at some other units, due to site restrictions.

-     The Middlesex Hospital's clinical and medical oncology services, with their high level of laboratory based development, are substantially bigger than those at the Royal Free Unit. The re-location cost of the Royal Free Unit moving to the Middlesex would be appreciably lower than that of the Middlesex Departments moving to the Royal Free. (Much of the space is University owned and financed by cancer research organisations, which given the current funding situation of these organisations is a further reason for concentrating services on the Middlesex site).

(vii)   The Middlesex Hospital has the stronger support services, its imaging department, adjacent to the radiotherapy department, has two MRIs and one CT. A particularly well developed Academic Department of nuclear medicine and considerable specialisation in pathology services is directed towards cancer, again both located close to the oncology service areas.

-     The UCH/Middlesex Centre also has a greater concentration of specialist services/facilities:-

-     A dedicated adolescent unit.

-     An Academic Department in Plastic Surgery.

-     A supra-Regional service for certain bone tumours, in conjunction with the Royal National Orthopaedic Hospital.

-     The CRC Counselling and Communication in Cancer Unit (recently moved from Whitechapel).

-     The relatively close proximity of the Hospital for Sick Children at Great Ormond Street to the Middlesex Unit (under I mile) compared with the Royal Free, means that the support for aspects of paediatric oncology, already much developed, could be continued without disruption. This might also include the supra-Regional retinoblastoma service now at St. Bartholomew's, although there may well be other suitable hospitals.

- The Middlesex Hospital has a wider range of specialties relevant to providing a high quality service for cancer patients, including plastic surgery, oral surgery and the St. Peter's Urology Group. The amalgamation of the Royal National Throat, Nose and Ear Hospital onto the Middlesex site provides a focus for an exceptional level of expertise in head and neck cancer.

(viii) The conclusion of the Review Group's analysis is that in service terms the weight of advantage for a major cancer centre lies with the UCH/Middlesex Unit.

Research and Development

(ix) The cancer research at the Middlesex/UCH in association with University College, is very highly regarded in national terms. It is substantial in volume and wide ranging, from basic science and molecular medicine to clinical research and development. Strong research activity is found in surgical, clinical and medical oncology. Recent investment in research here has totalled £l6M, a much greater investment than at the Royal Free.

(x) The other consideration in favour of the UCH/Middlesex site is its proximity to the exceptionally strong basic science facilities and research groups of University College. The advice from Cancer Research Organisations is that they are keen to make further investment in research on the UCH/Middlesex site in association with University College.

(xi) All the advice received by the Review Group in examining the quality and future potential of R & D for cancer, has confirmed that the association between UCH/Middlesex Hospital and University College London represents, one of the strongest research partnerships in the capital.

(xii) Whilst there is also excellent academic oncology and haematology at the Royal Free, it is of considerably smaller volume than that at UCH/Middlesex. There is some similarity in the content of the research in the two hospitals. It is known that on the medical oncology side, the research groups have already indicated a desire to bring their activities together onto one site, if possible.

7.6.7 Conclusions

(i) If the North Middlesex is to continue (and expand to meet the needs of a large population outside inner London as we propose: see section 8), the balance of argument we believe favours centralisation of radiotherapy and medical oncology services at the Middlesex/UCH from the Royal Free site.

(ii)   The position should be worked towards, over the next 3-4 years, by careful planning between the two hospitals, in conjunction with existing plans for the medical schools to link more closely together.

(iii)   This re-location from the Royal Free Hospital will certainly not call into question the Trust's overall future. The impact will however need effective management as cancer services leaving aside Haematology currently contribute less than 3% of the overall income of the unit.

(iv)   The relocation of recently (charitably) funded medical oncology services of the Royal Free to UCH/Middlesex would have some capital costs, £1M has been our order of magnitude figure, this would be considerably smaller than costs incurred in re-locating radiotherapy from the Middlesex to the Royal Free.

(v)   Should the review of acute hospitals in outer London indicate that the North Middlesex Hospital would not be an appropriate siting for an expansion of specialist cancer services, which is the preference of the Review, then the options of maintaining (and expanding) services at the Royal Free, as against a substantial capital spend, possibly involving a complete re-location of the service from Middlesex to UCH, would need to be examined. The Review Team believe that given the substantial capital investment made in cancer treatment facilities and other services on the Middlesex site in recent years, a particularly strong case would need to be made for a further relocation back to the UCH site.

(vi)   It is envisaged that the Royal Free will continue to have a large Haematology Unit but without on-site radiotherapy. The development of high dose chemotherapy for solid tumours may well be best concentrated on the Middlesex site.

(vii)   The two medical oncology units could merge relatively quickly say by April 1995 in the vacant university space within the existing oncology research area at the Middlesex site. Some 25 extra beds are expected to be required on the Middlesex site, for the overall transferred service. This we were assured could be accommodated.

(viii) The area for expanding the Middlesex Radiotherapy Department has been identified and although the costs would be quite high, the unit has already had experience of creating good quality adaptations within the department.

(ix)   The two medical schools will need to be drawn together to progress this merger plan, given their needs for staffing, space and research organisation.

(x)   It is envisaged that the enlarged Centre at the Middlesex would serve a population of approximately I.IM and would require facilities to serve a population of 3,600 new clinical/medical oncology patients per annum. The capital investment required would be of the order of £2.5-£3M.

(xi)   Whilst the Royal Free Hospital would lose its on-site radiotherapy and some medical oncology if our proposals are followed, it would still require a substantial oncology service by outreach from the Middlesex/UCH. The arrangements should be similar to those that will need to obtain at St. George's, King's, and St. Mary's hospitals, and should strengthen the existing arrangements by adding all the advantages in both service and research terms of the skills and facilities of a large cancer centre, to an appropriate on-site consultative presence.

(xii)   It should considerably strengthen the combined cancer services of the Royal Free and UCH/Middlesex for the future.

7.7 FUTURE PATTERN OF SPECIALIST HAEMATOLOGY SERVICES

7.7.1 A suggested arrangement in London

Local and secondary referral services in haematology related to malignant disease will be required at the most of the main teaching hospitals and local acute hospitals in and around London.

Tertiary services should, on advice given to the Review Group and its considered view, only be offered on a similar number of sites to that proposed for cancer centres; at most five in central London. Where possible these sites should be the same for both services.

It is therefore proposed that there should be some four centres in total at

> UCH/Royal Free
> The Royal London/St. Bartholomew's
> Guy's/St. Thomas'/King's
> Charing Cross/Hammersmith.

Outside London services would continue at the Royal Marsden (Sutton), linked with St. Georges.

As to the actual hospital in each group in which the services come to be based, we propose that discussions should take place at clinical and management level, with the view to coordination of these services through a careful and planned process and change. Changes in patient flow, stemming from the health service market, will be an important factor in these discussions.

It has been observed at our visits, that clinical haemato-oncology at various levels of intensity, is being carried out at almost all of the Centres we have seen. We have not been able within our timescale, and without having clinical haematology advice on the Review Group, to go into the detail required to make proposals we consider sound - or more than general - for either the Central London hospitals or those outside London. We therefore suggest that a separate small group should undertake such a study. It should be led by a clinical haematologist from outside the Thames Regions, who's name might be put forward jointly by the Royal Colleges of Pathologists and Physicians. It might be appropriate to undertake this study when final decisions on the future location of the major London cancer centres are known.

8.1 INTRODUCTION

Four units; North Middlesex Hospital, Oldchurch Hospital (Romford), the Sutton branch of the Royal Marsden Hospital and Mount Vernon Hospital, lie close to or outside the North/South Circular, but are inside the M.25. They vary in terms of their size, the quality of their facilities, the extent to which they are involved in research and the extent to which they serve populations that would not otherwise have reasonable access to a Specialist Centre.

Before examining these four units, we also give some consideration to the six other NHS units that lie outside the M25 but are still within the Thames Regions, and to the Reading and Northampton Centres in the Oxford Region, since changes in referral patterns to and from these will have consequences for the 'inner ring' Centres.

8.2 CENTRES OUTSIDE THE M25

South of the Thames

8.2.1 Maidstone Unit

(i) This was reported to be the only completely new oncology centre built in England in the last 20 years; it opened in April this year at a cost of £23m. It sets a design standard which future capital investment for cancer services should seek to emulate, and the effectiveness of which, in use, should be carefully audited so as to inform future provision in other places.

(ii) The 1992/3 workload of the unit is expected to be 2,000 new clinical/ medical oncology patients. The Review Group expects this to rise somewhat faster than previous estimates to over 3,000 new registered patients within two years. The Unit is designed to serve a 1.2m population.

(iii) Full utilisation of the excellent facilities of the Unit is likely to become constrained by the throughput limit of the three Linacs. An additional bunker, or pair thereof, could be added to the Department without disrupting its operation or the quality of functional relationships with other parts of the Centre. This would ensure that the major capital investment already made is fully exploited. It could be achieved at moderate cost in this open site, and without disruption of service.

(iv)   We recommend that the South East Thames RHA and local Health Authorities should review the DGHs to which the Maidstone Unit could be linked by <u>June 1994</u> to allow a timely decision vis-a-vis additional equipment capacity being needed. As the Consultants spend 1 ½ days a week out of the Centre already, there is limited scope to widen the network of linked DGHs without an extra consultant, the cost of which might well be supported by the business plan.

(v)   As the Oncology Unit has so recently moved onto the established DGH site, the development of joint working with surgical colleagues is at an early stage. The Medical Director and his colleagues are moving quickly to consolidate a clearer pattern of sub-specialisation within the Oncology group itself, and with the surgeons, as well as completing the planned development of protocols.

(vi)   The new Unit has attracted good calibre senior physics and radiography staff, and it will be important to achieve the same in terms of medical staff with appropriate special interests, as the Centre develops to full capacity.

(vii)   Local clinicians, managers and other members of the oncology team recognise that a major staff development programme is needed, linked to the rapid introduction of clinical audit systems. These measures are needed to create a new unified department from the two previous ones (Rochester and Pembury), and to ensure the sophisticated range of equipment is used to its full potential.

(viii)   Since the more distant areas served, (Hastings and Eastbourne) are some 40 miles away from the Centre, consideration should be given to increasing the small proportion of hostel beds and creating some hotel beds.

(ix)   There would be benefits to both the Canterbury Cancer Centre and that at Maidstone, in closer links being developed between them. Areas where this could be mutually helpful are cross cover in instances of radiography and physics staff shortages, staff training and possible rotational schemes, joint protocol development and review, co-ordinated audit and other professional development activities. This would also allow support to be given from Maidstone when serious equipment breakdown or replacement would (as recently) much impair the capacity, of the small centre in Canterbury to work to the best advantage.

8.2.2 Canterbury Unit

(i)   Given that the travel times to London Centres for the population served by this unit exceed those set by the Review, only limited comments on this Unit seem relevant to our remit. Set in a 400 bed DGH, the Unit treated 1700 new patients in 1992 and serves a population in East Kent of some 650,000 people.

(ii)   The Unit is unlikely, due to its geographical location, to significantly increase in size. To overcome the inherent limitations of this situation, it is recommended that closer ties are developed with the new Maidstone Unit as described previously.

8.2.3 Brighton Unit

(i)   This Unit, with some 2,000 new patients per annum, is located on the edge of the main Royal Sussex County Hospital site. The staff of the Unit are concerned that the hillside location makes expansion of the unit difficult to achieve. The space-constrained facilities have been partially modernised and extended predominantly through local fund raising efforts, in a cost-effective manner.

(ii)   Although the Unit only serves a population of some 750,000 the predominance of old people means the demand for services is substantially more, as evidenced by the workload. A fourth consultant has recently been appointed to bring the previously excessive workload into line with the average for other outer London Centres.

(iii)   The Unit was well organised in terms of tumour specialisation, within the limits of the small group of consultants. A highly efficient service exists with outreach clinics often held jointly with other specialties. A range of protocols and a well developed network of hospices all combine to allow the unit to run with only II beds, although this number is likely to be increased we understand. Another pressure point of the Unit has been the existence of a single Linac. This is now being remedied with an additional machine being commissioned at present.

(iv)   The Cancer Service benefits by there being a high level of surgical sub-specialisation.

(v)   The Unit serves a population covering Eastbourne, Haywards Heath and Worthing as well as Brighton itself, and has well organised patient transport arrangements. There is only a minimal referral rate to London, mostly for very rare cancers.

(vi)   The overall impression was of a well organised Unit which was working with inherent site difficulties, and a low level of capital investment made in recent years, apart from effective local fund-raising. The Department showed a high level of clinical organisation and an extremely efficient use of resources.

(vii)   The Review Group has concluded that this Centre will remain, serving a discrete population with a high proportion of elderly people. It would therefore be sensible for a long term site development plan for the Cancer Unit to be worked out, since any further expansion on the present site would be extremely expensive. An undercover access from the radiotherapy Centre to the adjacent main hospital, not involving the present walk up a public road on a steep hill, would seem an urgent need, especially for elderly patients.

8.2.4 Midhurst Unit

(i)   This 150 bed private hospital with charitable status, includes a small Cancer Treatment Unit, established some 13 years ago, which has one Linac and one superficial radiotherapy machine, plus a simulator and planning unit. CT and MRI are on site. The main population served is to the South of the Unit. The consultants, who visit the Unit, are from Guildford, Portsmouth and Southampton. The Unit runs as a satellite of the Guildford Unit in terms of support services, apart from the physicist input which is provided by the Cromwell.

(ii)   Cancer Services form a small part of the overall NHS workload. The presence of this Unit has little or no impact on the pattern of services in London, so that the Review Team has not assessed it in any further depth.

8.2.5 Reading Unit

(i)   This was the only Cancer Centre visited during the Review that lies outside the Thames Regions. The Unit currently serves approximately ½M people, and has some 1200 new patients per annum, shared between the two existing consultants. There is a relatively weak set of DGH links, but clear opportunities for a wider population to be served more conveniently by the Unit, than through current referral patterns. It would seem likely that the Unit will become the principal Centre for most of Berkshire's population. The Unit now has excellent quality facilities, following an imaginative modernisation scheme costing £3.5M, half of which was raised by local contributions. The refurbishment of the Department has achieved remarkable value for money, with an attractive design created within a listed building.

(ii)   A second Linac is being commissioned, and a spare bunker exists, as well as other equipment needed for an expanded workload. The Unit has 13 beds, with three hospices within the immediate catchment area. Day Unit and hostel beds are planned.

(iii)   The conclusions of the Review Group were that this Unit was likely to absorb referrals that currently go to a number of London Hospitals, including Mount Vernon and Hammersmith Hospitals. This would require an additional consultant to be appointed, and would be a cost effective use of these good facilities, and probably supported by a business plan.

8.2.6 Guildford Unit

(i)   The centre is located within 10 minutes of the M25 and on the A3, and so is accessible to a large population living in South West London. Approximately 60% of the hospital's patients comes from areas closer to London. The areas covered include Redhill, Farnham, Weybridge, Chertsey, Crawley and Camberley.

(ii)   In recent years almost all acute services apart from the Cancer Unit have been relocated from the St. Luke's site onto the large modern and attractively designed main Royal Surrey County Hospital site at Guildford. A £12M scheme has begun that will be completed in 1995, and provide a comprehensive Cancer Centre with an adjacent MRI unit already in place, and with ward accommodation being conveniently located in an adjacent modern main block of the hospital.

(iii)   The new unit is designed to serve a population of 1.2/1.3M. The main facilities will be 4 radiotherapy bunkers with 3 Linacs being initially installed (transferred from the existing site), plus other equipment for this size of unit.

(iv)   The Unit already has five consultants, and a sixth is proposed as a joint academic appointment with the University of Surrey. The new unit will have approximately 50 beds (no hostel or hotel beds are currently proposed).

(v)   Site specialisation has been a long standing characteristic of the unit with the lead consultant having responsibility for creating and updating protocols for their area of expertise, which other consultants then follow.

(vi)   Consultants from the unit spend three sessions a week at Frimley Hospital, one at Chertsey, two at Redhill and two at Crawley, as well as three sessions being held at Midhurst.

(vii)   The Unit has had a strong tradition of surgical specialisation, in oncology with two of the six surgeons specialising in colo-rectal cancer. One breast surgeon links with the breast screening centre which is on site. There are also specialist units in Maxillo facial and ENT surgery within the Hospital.

(viii)   The Unit already has strong links with Surrey University which is adjacent to the main hospital, for example in bio-engineering, physics. (MRI research), bio-chemistry and micro-biology. A network of joint appointments is planned that will further strengthen this relationship. A breast cancer group is already based at Surrey University funded by the ICRF. There are also gynaecological research links, and expertise of international standing in analyzing tumour response to treatment.

(ix)   The Review Group sees the planned development on the Royal Surrey site as a well-placed out of London Centre, which is likely to expand beyond the initial equipment capacity once the new unit is established. Travel times would suggest that part of the Basingstoke area, as well as some areas closer to London, could look to this centre in the longer term. We believe that there should also be close links between this unit and the Royal Marsden at Sutton.

North of the Thames

8.2.7 A new unit in North West Thames?

(i)   This situation is less satisfactory than the Southern picture. The North West of London does not have a single unit outside the M25, despite the large population along the M1 towards Birmingham. Mount Vernon is an accessible Centre by road, with a travel time of well under an hour, for a substantial population but poorly served by public transport. However some localities which the hospital serves, are around an hour's travel time away, and the Review Team believes that consideration should be given to how best the northern part of this population should be best served. From the information available it is unlikely that a large enough population of North West Thames Region would use such a new unit to justify a modern Centre being created.

(ii)   The Review Group would be concerned if a further small Centre were to be built anywhere in the South East of England. The Lister Hospital Trust at Stevenage recognises the uneconomic size of a previously proposed unit (resulting in a weak investment/business plan for the new unit). The compromise proposal to reduce capital costs by treatment planning being carried out at Mount Vernon for a satellite treatment unit at Stevenage is not regarded as an appropriate way of developing a new service. It would create unnecessary difficulties in quality control.

(iii)   The Review believes that a review should be undertaken by North West Thames, Oxford and East Anglia Regions, as to how best patients in the areas of Bedford, Milton Keynes, Luton, Stevenage and Hitchin should be served. The Centre at Northampton is currently small, and has expansion capacity. This option, and that of a new Centre of adequate size at for instance Luton or Stevenage, require evaluation. In the Review Group's view, such an evaluation should have been completed no later than December 1993.

To the North East of London the service provision, outside the M25, is by two small units at Colchester and Southend.

8.2.8 The Colchester Unit

(i)   The Unit's facilities are of mixed quality, better than those seen at Oldchurch and Canterbury, but inferior to those at Southend, let alone the exceptional standards recently created at Maidstone.

(ii)   The Colchester Cancer Unit will be the only acute service left on the Essex County Hospital site by the end of the year; the DGH services having been concentrated on Colchester General Hospital site. The senior staff of the Cancer Unit confirmed that it cannot stay on its existing site, and that it would clearly be a poor investment therefore to spend £1.5M to remedy the immediate physical shortcomings of the Unit. There is an urgent need to decide on the future location of a replacement Centre. The Review Team were impressed by the professional commitment of local clinicians and their willingness to relocate if a larger Unit could be created that would be able to provide a better service. The key advantages they would wish to see achieved would be:-

-    A larger grouping of Consultants, allowing greater site specialisation.

-    Co-location with general DGH services.

-    Better research support.

-    A complete range of modern equipment being available, as well as stronger physics, radiography and pharmacy support.

-    An appropriate level of nurse specialists and other support staff.

(iii)   The Review has concluded that the future of the Colchester service needs to be considered together with the Oldchurch Unit, which also needs to be replaced within a short time scale (see below). Whilst it is not for this Review of medical services in London to suggest a site, we do believe that Chelmsford could have many advantages.

(iv)   Whatever the outcome of such an evaluation, it is important that the high level of Oncology expertise available to local Consultants, GPs and the population in and around Colchester be preserved.

8.2.9 Southend Unit

(i)   This Unit has had recent investment, including a spacious well designed extra (3rd) linac suite and new ward facilities are to be constructed close to the Radiotherapy Department. A modern CT suite is also conveniently close for treatment planning.

(ii)   The service offered is well organised with a good level of co-ordinated working with local DGHs and primary care services, including hospices. Multi-disciplinary management of cancer involving surgeons as well as oncologists was also evident. The Unit provides an economic as well as a good quality service.

(iii)   The Centre serves a relatively small, distinctly defined population (700,000), and has a small network of linked DGHs with which it plans to work even more closely by consultants spending up to three days a week per site. The opportunity of the Unit to serve a larger population and so treat more than the current 2,000 new clinical/medical oncology patients per annum is limited. This creates inherent drawbacks for the further development of the cancer service.

(iv)   To partly overcome these problems the Review Team strongly support the local plans for the links between the Colchester and Southend Units being strengthened, to their mutual benefit. (The arrangements should be similar to those previously described for the Canterbury and Maidstone Units.

8.3   CENTRES IN OUTER LONDON

(i)   The Review Group supports the continued existence of a pattern of Specialist Cancer Centres in outer London, where substantial populations live. Such Centres offer some advantages in terms of access compared with inner London Units - less traffic congestion, easier car parking, and better developed community support in many instances, (for example volunteer car drivers). However public transport links are often less well developed to serve a large population than for some inner London Centres. Operating costs are usually lower and so such Units have the prospect of providing more economic services. Such outer London Units are often also on more spacious sites than inner London, and can be expanded with less cost.

(ii)   While there is a widespread understanding that the number of acute hospitals in inner London will reduce, the two North Thames Regions have told us that the current pattern of hospitals in outer London is also unlikely to be sustainable.

(iii)   The Review Group acknowledges that the future location of specialist Cancer Centres in outer London will have to be resolved within the future pattern of acute hospitals overall.

(iv)   The Review has concentrated its assessment of the outer London Units to an examination of the range and quality of the existing cancer facilities and services, and their future prospects, but does not have the information to take into account any possible whole hospital relocations outside London.

8.3.1 The North Middlesex Unit

(i)   This Centre is modern, with well laid out facilities that form a coherent unit. Furthermore, of all the 21 sites visited, it offered amongst the most straight forward and economical opportunities to virtually double the existing capacity of the Unit, yet still retain a contiguous set of wards, radiotherapy department, clinic and chemotherapy day facilities. The Unit has the potential to provide a high quality service to a larger population than is currently the case. (Expansion of the Pathology and Imaging Departments will be less straightforward).

(ii)   The Centre provides a well organised service. 70% of new patients are seen in DGH outreach clinics. The three Consultants spend one day a week in linked DGHs. There is a good level of surgical commitment to oncology. It is however a small unit (1,437 new clinical/medical oncology patients in 91/2) and will need to grow to provide a comprehensive service for the future. The Review Group recommend a more modest initial expansion to allow the unit to serve 2,500 to 3,000 new patients p.a., which would cost £3M.

(iii)   The North Middlesex Hospital is located with good access to the M25 and M11, giving it reasonable access from parts of Hertfordshire and Essex which one well within the travel time limit of one hour. The Unit could therefore expect to expand in size by establishing a wider network of linked DGHs associated with the proposed relocation of other existing Units, both in London and at Oldchurch.

(iv)   The management and clinical staff appeared well integrated and committed to improving as well as expanding the service provided.

(v)   The weaknesses of the Unit are:-

-       Its small size.

-       The limited extent of sub-specialisation possible amongst the small group of oncologists.

-       The lack of strategic clarity about the acute hospital pattern in this part of North London.

(vi)   The Review Team have concluded that the siting of the North Middlesex, the quality of its facilities, and their ease of expansion, combined with the good organisation the hospital displayed, all point to, in the particular context of cancer services, it being expanded.

(vii)   This plan has to be assessed within the overall future pattern of acute services in this part of north London.

8.3.2 Oldchurch Hospital

(i)   This Centre is the smallest of the four in the outer London ring, with some 1232 new clinical/medical oncology patients in 1991/2 drawn from a more localised catchment area than the others. 77% of the patients come from within the Barking, Havering and Brentwood Health Authority.

(ii)   The hospital is part of a split site acute unit, the other half being Harold Wood Hospital on the other side of Romford. The Trust is considering as a matter of urgency how to centralise services on one site. The facilities of the Cancer Centre were poor reflecting the prolonged periods of previous uncertainty about the Unit's future (The closure of the Unit was first proposed in 1979). The local DHA supported its relocation to the Harold Wood site when its closure was proposed in 1987. Harold Wood Hospital has for some years had outreach oncology services from the London Hospital, which we have been told that they wish to continue, and which the London are certainly willing to continue.

(iii)   Staff locally acknowledged the need to achieve a 'minimum critical mass' of 3,000 + new patients per annum for the Unit to have an assured future. However, it was clear that such a development would be difficult to achieve, except by a completely new build. (If the Trust were to decide not to redevelop the Oldchurch site, but concentrate services at Harold Wood Hospital, then a complete new build would obviously be required in any case, but there still would not seem to be a large enough number of patients to support this.

(iv)   The Review Group has concluded that the existing services should be relocated, given:-

-       The poor quality facilities.

-       The restricted range of on site general hospital services, and of oncology sub-specialisation.

-       Present and future recruitment difficulties for physicists and radiographers.

-       The high cost of re-development on its existing site;

-       The unlikelihood of the Unit achieving the size regarded as the minimum for a good quality, cost-effective service in the future.

(v)   However, both Harold Wood and Oldchurch Hospital (while it remains in use) should retain a strong DGH oncology presence even if the Specialist Centre is not retained.

(vi)   It is anticipated from an analysis of travel times, that the following existing Units would receive extra patients: The Royal London hospital, North Middlesex and Colchester or Southend. They already have the capacity to care for the 1,232 new clinical/medical oncology patients without the delay of a significant capital investment being required.

(vii)   We recommend that the North East Thames R.H.A., with the relevant local Health Authorities, should immediately set up a review to identify whether the rebuilding of two small Centres at Colchester and Oldchurch can be justified in capital investment terms, and more importantly service quality terms, as opposed to a single, more comprehensive Centre being built. The view of the Review Group is that people in Essex would benefit more by having a single, centrally located Centre of similar quality to those at Maidstone or Guildford, possibly at Chelmsford.

8.3.3 The Sutton Branch of the Royal Marsden Hospital

(i)   Although not particularly well served by public transport (Sutton Station is ten minutes by bus - the M25 is a ten minute drive away), the Unit is nevertheless the most conveniently placed centre for a sizeable population in Surrey and South London.

(ii)   The site is some ten times bigger than that at Fulham Road and has had a range of good quality developments that form a well laid out set of facilities. The Radiotherapy Centre is an excellent example, like Mount Vernon and Charing Cross, of how a large Unit can avoid being impersonal or oppressive. The Department has four modern Linacs, a spare bunker and two Cobalt Unit. (There is also a total body radiation machine remote from the main department).

(iii)   The day unit, chemotherapy area and palliative care ward all provide excellent quality physical facilities, and the nursing and other professional staff were clearly highly organised and committed; reflecting the national standing of the hospital for specialist nurse training. 75% of the chemotherapy workload of the Royal Marsden is carried out at Sutton.

(iv)   The Sutton site has a large and varied research role with particularly important research in physics and in new cancer drug development.

(v)   St. George's is six miles away and there is already a range of established shared consultant posts (reflected in the £250k paid for medical staffing support provided by St. George's). The St. George's medical staff are keen to extend the collaborative work with the Sutton Unit.

(vi)   The Review Team believes there would be clear advantages for the population of this area of South London and parts of Surrey, if the Sutton branch of the Royal Marsden Hospital is expanded to provide a more comprehensive local service including gynaecology, and head and neck cancer services.

(vii)   The two main limitations of this plan are that the Sutton Branch of the Royal Marsden Hospital is:-

-       An isolated single specialty unit.

-       Has a limited surgical capacity (one theatre), without on-site, 24 hour surgical cover.

(viii) The drawbacks of its single specialty situation, can be minimised by further improving the service and management links with St. George's:-

-       The level of surgical sub-specialisation for particular tumour areas could be improved. Complex cancer surgery, requiring the facilities of a major teaching hospital with I.T.U., out of hours theatre and pathology teams, could be carried out at the St. George's site, rather than people having to travel into central London.

-       Joint appointments between St. George's and the Sutton branch of the Marsden will allow a higher level of co-ordinated surgical, radiotherapy and oncology care to be provided, than a more distant link with a large acute unit in Central London could achieve. The continued linkage with the Fulham Road Branch of the Marsden cannot overcome this problem as the required clinical expertise is not available from that location.

-       The new paediatric unit (a £4.24m charitably funded development) would benefit from more close involvement with St. George's Hospital's considerable range of children's expertise. This will be subject to the views of the Specialty Children's Services Review.

(ix)   The lack of continuity of patient care caused by medical staff covering up to three NHS sites could be improved if appointments cease to be split three ways, covering the two Royal Marsden Branches and an undergraduate teaching hospital as well. The proposed links with St. George's will still involve split site working, but it will be between two rather than three sites which are only six rather than 15 miles apart.

(x)   In the Review Group's view the overall potential of the Sutton branch of the Royal Marsden seems most likely to be best developed, and its limitations minimised by its management being joined with that of St. George's. It is recommended that this take place from 1st April 1994. This merger will benefit both institutions:

-       The Royal Marsden (Sutton Branch) gaining a more full time presence from a wider range of surgical, general medical and paediatric consultants, and other junior staff, than the current arrangement which the Royal Marsden (Fulham Road) can offer.

-       St. George's will gain by the proposed expansion of the Royal Marsden (Sutton Branch) providing locally a more comprehensive cancer treatment service, and by some consultants not working on three sites (both of these of the Marsden and St. George's) any longer.

-       The opportunities for co-ordinated research between the two institutions will be improved (St. George's is unusual in having two full time medical oncologists already with established research interests).

-       The St. George's undergraduates will gain by the closer association of the two institutions, as will postgraduate training programmes of both hospitals.

-       Most importantly people living in a large area of South London and parts of Surrey, will benefit from the expansion with the Sutton Branch of the Marsden providing a more complete, locally accessible service than is currently available.

8.3.4 Mount Vernon

(i)   Mount Vernon is the largest centre in South East England and demonstrates many of the advantages which the Review is seeking to achieve by more comprehensive Units being created across London. An extended description of its facilities is given below as they address many of the doubts about creating larger Centres.

-       This large Centre demonstrates how a service with over 5,000 new cases registered per annum, can avoid being impersonal. The well thought out design of the five Linac radiotherapy department, with a number of separate waiting areas, in close contact with small groups of staff, is a good model.

-       A sustained patient focused approach to care is evident in a high quality ten bedroom hotel unit, and the new complementary therapy and patient information and support unit. The extended working day and availability of services at weekends, covered by voluntary overtime, centred on the CHART research programme, has allowed more flexibility for patients about their treatment times. (Young breast cancer patients have in particular used the early and late bookings). These arrangements also produce more effective use of expensive equipment. This initiative should be examined by other units.

-       The Mount Vernon Unit has exceptionally well developed links with a number of DGHs, with consultants spending up to half their working week in these local hospitals.

- A substantial level of tumour site specialisation exists amongst the large group of consultants.

- Experienced senior physiotherapists and radiographers are in post who take a wide range of responsibilities, relieving medical staff of some duties within the Unit, as well as playing a wider regional role in developing improved staff training and quality control/assurance systems.

- An exceptional level of dedicated diagnostic facilities (2 MRI and a CT) show what such a large Unit can achieve while remaining cost-effective.

- A modern set of equipment and a fifth Linac are being installed. The replacement costs, in spite of the volume of equipment, are the lowest, projected up to 1999, of the 15 Units in London.

- The first combined CT/Simulator in southern England is being installed. (This should be the subject of a Health Technology Assessment exercise by the DoH as it not only reduces the number of times a patient has to attend for planning prior to treatment, but could also produce significant staff savings).

- A high level of research takes place relative to other non-teaching hospitals visited, now recognised in funding terms by the DoH (£1.3M). The substantial C.R.C. investment (80 staff) in the Gray Laboratory, which is one of the few U.K. research units that concentrates on radiobiology research and is sensibly located close by a large radiotherapy department. The staff in the centre lead in what may be a most important national research programme aimed to improve cure rates by radiation therapy (the CHART study).

- A well developed palliative care service is on site, with extensive outreach arrangements.

(ii) The principal current weaknesses which the Unit needs to address were seen to be:-

- The high workload of the consultants given their time commitments to DGHs.

- The relatively low level of specialist medical oncology input within the existing consultant group (one shared appointment only), although it is accepted that clinical oncologists often carry out a full range of oncology services.

- The limited extent of surgical sub-specialisation in different areas of oncology.

- There is a need to further strengthen the academic unit.

(iii) The future prospects of the Mount Vernon Unit will be influenced significantly by:-

- The proposed provision of more local oncology services in the North of the Region which could reduce the current Mount Vernon workload by up to some 10%. The impact of this change would be greater on the Northampton and Cambridge Units; in our opinion the former is already below an optimum size. To a lesser extent the likely increased flow of patients to Reading would also reduce the current size of the unit, but by less than 5%. The Reading Unit has recently received significant capital investment.

  The Oxford RHA and North West Thames with their respective local Health Authorities need to agree a timetable for reviewing the linkages of DGHs to both the Hammersmith and Mount Vernon Hospitals. This may also need to involve East Anglia Region because the catchment population in the neighbourhood of Bedford at present goes to Cambridge, although it is nearer to Northampton.

- The extent to which Mount Vernon retains a substantial surgical presence with greater specialisation in oncological work. (The unit currently lacks ENT and Gynaecology beds).

- The future pattern of acute units overall in North West London.

(iv) Overall the Review Group regard Mount Vernon as offering one of the best organised and most patient-sensitive services of those seen in the Review. The review of the overall future pattern of acute services in North West London will be completed by the end of the year, we are informed. This will therefore coincide with the review into whether a change of referral patterns in the North of the Region should be planned with a view to improving access for an increasingly aging population of patients with cancer.

9.1   PROJECTED SIZE AND WORKLOAD OF THE PROPOSED EIGHT
       SPECIALIST CANCER CENTRES

By analyzing existing patient referral data, examining anticipated DGH
linkages and taking increases in incidence into account, the following
future pattern has been calculated:

Projections for Proposed Cancer Centres in 1996/97	Projected Pop. Served* 000s	Total New Cancer Cases Generated by Pop.Served **	New Onc. Patients Treated at Centres ***	Proposed No.of Linacs Required ****
Guy's	1,251	5,443	3,992	6
Mount Vernon*	1,337	5,453	3,999	6
Charing Cross*	1,097	4,791	3,514	5
UCH/Middx.*	1,143	4,914	3,604	5
Nth.Middx.	885	3,375	2,475	4
Royal London	1,134	4,913	3,603	5
Royal Marsden, Sutton	1,064	4,534	3,325	5
Hammersmith*	703	2,867	2,103	3
Total London Centres	8,614	36,290	26,615	39
Total Non-London Thames Centres	5,743	26,179	19,198	
Grand Total Thames Centres	14,357	62,469	45,813	
Comparison with 1991/2 Projections	14,196	57,403	42,096	

*   Includes Notional Population for inflows from Oxford Region.

**   Based on Thames Cancer Registry Incidence data (excluding non-
        melanoma skin) for each DHA proposed to be served by the Centre,
        OPCS 1996 Population estimates and a projected cancer incidence
        increase of 7.50% for the five years between 1991 and 1996.

***   New patients treated allow for an estimated 10% under-registration of
        patients by the Thames Cancer Registry and are based on the Review
        Group's assessment that two thirds of all new cancer cases will at some

point be treated in a Specialist Cancer Centre. The ratio of new cancer cases to new patients treated in the current London Centres has been difficult to derive because of different protocols for counting new patients at the current Centres (see section 5.4 of the report).

**** Estimates of machine requirements have been based on model utilisation rates agreed by the Review Group. In some cases it may be possible to reduce the number of machines based on more detailed local analysis of demand, machine utilisation and working practices, after taking account of the impact of Teaching, Research & Development.
Estates database indicates a current provision of 63 machines in the existing London Centres (40 linear accelerators, 13 cobalts and 10 deep x-ray machines).

9.2 ACCESSIBILITY

For the proposed centres, the population of the districts served in full or in part fall within the drive times as indicated below * :-

Centre	Rush hour 30 mins	Rush hour 60 mins	Normal 30 mins	Normal 60 mins
Guy's	39%	80%	68%	100%
Mount Vernon	12%	52%	32%	100%
Charing Cross	58%	100%	96%	100%
UCH/Middlesex	59%	100%	98%	100%
North Middlesex	28%	62%	53%	75% **
Royal London	32%	57%	53%	84% **
Royal Marsden, Sutton	27%	78%	65%	100%
Hammersmith	71%	98%	98%	100%

* Information supplied by the London Implementation Group
** To be further assessed by reviews by North Thames Regions regarding new centres being created.

From a comparison of public and private transport travel times, the difference is more marked for a 30 minute journey in favour of private transport. For 60 minute journeys with the differences become smaller.

9.3   THE PROJECTED SIZE OF OTHER UNITS IN SOUTH EAST ENGLAND

	Million
Total population to be served	14.3*
Population served by London Centres	8.6
Population to be served by other Centres in the South East	5.7

*   Apart from the significant patient flows from Oxford RHA which are included in this population figure (150,000 approximate population), other patient inflows have been assessed to be broadly balanced by outflows. All figures are based on 1996 OPCS projections.

Current and proposed population (millions) to be served by outer London centres

	Current	Proposed
Canterbury	0.65	0.7
Maidstone	1.0	1.2
Colchester	0.8	-
New Essex Centre	-	1.0
Southend	0.7	0.7
Brighton	0.75	0.8
Guildford	1.2	1.3
	5.1	5.7*

*   The increase of 600,000 in population served is mainly due to the projected new Essex Unit absorbing much of the work currently located at Oldchurch and the reversal of flows from London to the new Maidstone Unit.

9.4   REVENUE IMPLICATIONS

Approximately £118M income was received by the 15 Specialist Cancer Centres in London 1991/92. £43M (i.e. 36%) was expended at the Royal Marsden Hospitals, yet in service volume terms that hospital contributed, on a generous assessment of its workload, some 20% of the total. (Allowance obviously needs to be made, however, for the heavy teaching role which the Hospital carries out and for service costs of research not covered from other sources.) The concentration of the two branches of the Royal Marsden onto one site is likely to create the most substantial revenue saving, without diminishing patient services, of any of the changes proposed. Any other whole site closures achieved in part by the concentration of cancer services, would also make significant savings.

Our more conservative estimate is that the creation of the eight larger Centres we recommend will allow expenditure to be contained at its present level, in spite of the 15% increase in incidence over the next 10 years, assuming treatment modalities do not change sharply. A more ambitious but still realistic assumption using the rest of the U.K. as a benchmark would suggest a 5% revenue saving should be possible, i.e. some £6M per annum (leaving aside site closure savings). The National Pricing Costing Working Party concluded that some 30% of a unit's costs are fixed and so the consolidation of the Royal Marsden on to one site should save some £6M per annum, i.e. the general efficiency improvement and site rationalisation could say 10% of current overall expenditure. (Should other site closures result, further substantial savings would accrue).

9.5   STAFF

9.5.1 Medical staffing

(i)   Appendix 3 gives the staffing profile for each of the 15 units in London. The aggregate picture is as follows:

Medical Staffing: Consultants in non-surgical oncology

Population		Clinical Oncology		Medical Oncology	
England & Wales	London Centres	England & Wales	London Centres	England only	London Centres
51M	8.6M (17%)	240	51 (21%)	86*	23 (27%)

* England only

(ii)   The funding of consultant posts is complicated and principally involves three sources:

-    NHS funding
-    Government (non-NHS) funding (University, MRC)
-    Charitable funding, e.g. ICRF and Cancer Relief Macmillan Fund

(iii)   Overall, some 20% of all the above posts are funded from non-NHS sources. This varies considerably between hospitals. The Royal Free has

70% of its consultant oncology posts in this category, whereas the Royal London and Mount Vernon have under 5% so funded.

(iv)   Estimates of the costs of consultant posts is further complicated by the difficulty of establishing whether a post is primarily a service position, a research post or, quite commonly, a combination of the two. Teaching also takes up a much greater part of the workload for some posts than for others. There is also the question of part time work and private practice. Where conducted off-site, we believe that private practice in London can significantly reduce consultant input in all branches of oncology.

(v)   The four Thames Regions currently have more oncology consultants for the population served than the England and Wales average. The Review Group believes that the grouping of consultants into a smaller number of units will not create redundancies, but instead will allow:-

-       Up to some four sessions per week to be spent by specialists in a local acute hospital(s).

-       Although cancer services are already a more 'consultant provided' service than many specialties, the existing number of consultants will need to be increased to implement 'Achieving a Balance' and the 'New Deal' for junior doctors, also, probably to meet the requirements of the Calman Report.

-       Greater sub-specialisation will be possible for individual clinicians.

-       A higher level of involvement of NHS staff in clinical research.

(vi)   We do not estimate that there will be any reduction in the 51 clinical oncologist posts of the London Units, but 16 will need to relocate to a different centre from the one in which they currently work. Similarly, the 23 medical oncologists should not suffer redundancies but 12 will need to relocate. These estimates do not take into account the changes described in the next paragraph.

Training Posts

(vii)   There are 56 registrar or senior registrar posts in the South East in clinical oncology and 20 in medical oncology (six posts now offer combined training which is a trend that we recommend should be extended). Unless current consultant numbers alter, the effect of JPAC will be that the number of clinical oncology training posts is likely to decline while the numbers in both medical oncology and palliative care are likely to increase.

(viii)   The more structured, shorter training proposed to the Calman Report (taken with changes in junior doctors' hours of work) and the effects of JPAC will, if accepted by the Government, reduce their service availability. Consultants will also have to spend more time training such junior staff. Of itself the proposed smaller number of larger specialist centres will enhance the breadth of training by the larger grouping of consultants present. Nevertheless, there will be implications for service cover here, which may well require more consultants and not just a transfer of senior registrars currently in training to consultant level posts.

9.5.2 Non-medical Staff

Therapeutic Radiographers

(i)   Some 269 whole time equivalent therapeutic radiographers work in the 15 London cancer centres. This represents 25% of the U.K. total. The profession is 97% female, with 44% being below 30 years of age. There are widespread recruitment problems within the Capital which accounts for 34% of total vacancies nationally.

(ii)   The total combined annual intake to the four Radiography Schools in the Thames Regions is around 50 places. This means that each of the schools is too small to make effective use of resources or develop sufficient specialised skills to train future generations of radiographers, in the view of the Review Team. In contrast, three Northern Health Regions have combined their training requirements into a single school based at Liverpool. The College of Radiographers favours extending such joint commissioning arrangements. The Review Team believes the four Thames Regions should consider such an approach. Part of this plan should also be to address the problem of the high drop-out rate during training, reported as being as high as 24% from a national survey carried out some four years ago, although we were told that it is now substantially lower. The four Thames Regions should, as part of this review, identify how retraining and refresher courses for qualified therapeutic radiographers can be made more available so that past investment made in their training is not lost unnecessarily, and that those that wish to return to work are encouraged to do so.

(iii)   There is room for further extension to the role of radiographers, such as taking on departmental management roles, specialist roles in information technology, quality assurance and in clinical co-ordination. These developments could be facilitated through relieving qualified staff of more routine duties by developing the use of helper grades and through changes in the way staff allocations and machines are organised.

(iv)   The significant reduction in megavoltage radiotherapy machines will have staffing implications which should be examined in conjunction with the possible longer hours of operation of equipment and the increasing complexity of quality control requirements. It is not possible to say as yet how the total staffing needed in the new arrangements we propose will differ from present levels. But no significant reduction is thought likely. It needs to be remembered that there is some shortage of radiographers nationally and a quite high staff turnover rate, so any minor reductions should be relatively easily managed.

Physicists

(v)   There are 71 whole time equivalent posts in the 15 London cancer centres. The four Thames Regions fund 9 training posts in medical physics per annum, of which 20%, i.e. two per year, are likely to specialise in radiotherapy. This scheme was set up a year or two ago as a response to long standing recruitment problems.

(vi)   The existing 71 WTE posts appear higher than needed in the future, as there would only be some 39 megavoltage treatment machines, rather than the 63 (megavoltage and deep X-Ray) machines which exist at present. It is appreciated, however, that medical physicists, including those who work for much of their time in radiotherapy also often have wider responsibilities outside this field. Their duties include those of radiation safety in other departments, of physical measurement in medicine, and others. In radiotherapy itself, the growing complexity of equipment and the accepted need for stricter quality assurance will require enough physicists to ensure that patients are treated to high standards. On the other hand, some changes in skill mix could well lead to a marginal reduction in the need for qualified physicists. Overall, we have concluded that the number of posts needed, if our recommendations are fully implemented, will be somewhat fewer than at present, but that given the difficulty in recruiting and retaining this group of staff, with consequent shortages into other centres, no redundancies are likely.

(vii)   Without creating a smaller number of Centres, there would be an increase in the number of staff required, who could well not be available, hence leading to risks of quality control and safety standards being compromised.

Nurses

(viii) Approximately 800 full time equivalent nursing posts were reported in our survey as working in the 15 London cancer centres. The variations in the number of nurses associated with different units was surprisingly wide and the Review Group therefore sought confirmation of the figures. This process has narrowed the original variation to an extent, but it nevertheless remains considerable. It is probably explained in part by the different case-mix of the units and in the extent to which surgical oncology is counted in.

Anticipated changes in oncology nursing

(ix)   There are already trends changing the work of nurses and in the number of different types of nurses required. In oncology nursing we believe that in the future, the principal developments are likely to be:

- A smaller proportion of the nursing workforce in cancer services being ward based. (Reflecting the development of a higher proportion of day treatments, the creation of hotel and hostel beds, a larger proportion of care being provided in local acute hospitals and the continued development of palliative care services outside specialist cancer centres).

- An increasing proportion of nurses will be specialists and provide outreach services to local general hospitals and primary care services, while being based in Specialist Cancer Centres.

- The proportion and absolute numbers of nurses working in the community with specialist skills of cancer services will need to increase so that, for example, the wishes of most people to die in their own homes rather than in hospital, can be met. This requires effective clinical expertise so that symptom control and also social and psychological support can be provided by multi-disciplinary teams, including nurse specialists.

The diverse range of nursing roles

(x)   Nurses are involved in the care of cancer patients within the specialist cancer centre itself, in both general and specialist wards at DGHs, as practice nurses and within the community as district nurses, health visitors and hospice nurses. In addition, there are charity funded nurses working in hospitals and in the community, such as Macmillan nurses, Marie Curie Foundation nurses and CLIC (Cancer and Leukaemia in Childhood) nurses of whom brief details are given below.

(xi)   **Macmillan nurses** may work in either hospitals or the community and are trained to advise on pain relief, symptom control, provision of psychosocial support and are an education and teaching resource. Macmillan nurses are funded by the Cancer Relief Macmillan Fund for 2-3 years initially, after which financial responsibility for their employment falls to the NHS Trust or independent hospice.

(xii)   **Marie Curie Foundation nurses** can be Registered General Nurses, Enrolled Nurses or Nursing Auxiliaries funded jointly by the charity and the NHS, who give care to cancer patients at home.

(xiii)   **The CLIC Trust** funds paediatric-trained oncology nurses to work with children with cancer both in and outside hospital.

(xiv) The role of the nurse in cancer services covers the provision of both acute and palliative care. The two types of care are almost never mutually exclusive but may be mixed in different proportions within the nurse's role depending on a patient's needs and stage of treatment, and the care setting.

(xv) The pattern is now well established of oncology nurses who are specialists in the care of patients with cancer at specific sites, such as breast cancer and cancer of the head and neck. An increasing number of posts are being established in these areas and others such as lymphodema management as well as cancer chemotherapy and counselling. Skill levels in all areas can be expected to increase as nurses expand their role to provide an increasingly comprehensive service within the multi-disciplinary team.

(xvi) Within DGHs, most cancer patients are treated by general nurses whose training will have covered the relevant areas of patient communication (including breaking bad news and bereavement care), symptom and pain control and psychosocial support. However, it is essential that at least some nurses within DGHs add to their general training by some specialist post basic education in cancer services.

(xvii) Although nurses in all settings have some involvement in palliative care, there is a need to develop centres of excellence and innovation in this area which can then be generalised to all areas of cancer nursing work. Standards of good practice, education and support are currently provided by nurses and other professionals with specialist training, working as Macmillan nurses, hospice staff and members of hospital and community support teams. The pattern of the nurse specialist in palliative care should be adopted by all DGHs.

(xviii) Some aspects of palliative care (information and support, bereavement counselling) are shared by all professions involved in the delivery of cancer services. There is a rationale, therefore, for a multi-disciplinary approach to specialist training in this area.

Pharmacists

(xix) The Thames Regions employ 25% of the national total of hospital pharmacists.

(xx) The continuing expansion in the use of cytotoxic drugs in cancer therapy, couple with the special hazards to staff in their preparation and use, means that the number of pharmacists specialising in this field will need to increase. There is evidence that a higher proportion than at present of the duties carried out by pharmacists could be more economically performed by a range of less skilled grades.

(xxi) Local acute hospitals are carrying out an increasing range of chemotherapy and the Review Group believes that quality standards would be best developed by the specialist pharmacists from cancer centres having a role in protocol design and audit, as well as achieving economies by centralising production and providing drug information services.

(xxii) We do not see a reduction in pharmacist numbers arising from our proposals.

Other key staff groups

(xxiii) A number of other disciplines play an important role in the delivery of good quality cancer services, for example psychologists, occupational therapists, dietitians, physiotherapists and speech therapists. The role of each of these groups needs to be specifically defined at primary, secondary and tertiary levels so that a better co-ordinated service can be provided to individual patients in the future, within the desired multi-disciplinary care team.

(xxiv) We believe that the smaller number of larger centres that we propose will help to ensure that there is flexibility in provision of these services for cancer patients.

9.6 CAPITAL IMPLICATIONS

Note: all costs are indicative estimates

9.6.1 Equipment

If the existing 15 Units continued to exist, the anticipated equipment replacement costs up to 1998 would be:-

	£M
All 14 cobalt units to be replaced by Linacs	7.0
10 of 40 Linacs replaced	5.0
8 of 13 superficial treatment machines replaced	0.8
4 of 16 afterloading machines replaced	0.4
1 of 16 simulators replaced	0.4
TOTAL	**£13.6M**

(This is an underestimate, as some departments are not fully equipped at present).

By centralising on eight sites, only nine new linacs instead of 24 would need to be purchased; six existing machines would need to be moved.

Allowing for transfer costs at £75,000 per machine, the proposed pattern of Centres would save approximately £7M, as against the status quo.

At the eight proposed Centres, eleven new bunkers would be required (Guy's four, Royal London three, Mount Vernon two, Middlesex one, Charing Cross one). This will cost in the region of £6.0M.

Some radiotherapy departments will need modernising to achieve the higher standard we propose for patients and staff. This is particularly true at Guy's and the Royal London, where the option of a substantially remodelled department would in each case need to be considered. We have allowed the sum of £5M at the Royal London and £4M at Guy's for these more major schemes. The Hammersmith, Middlesex, Royal Marsden (Sutton) and North Middlesex would need more minor capital expenditure on their radiotherapy departments, perhaps £3M in total. Further detail is to be found in our comments in section 7 on each centre.

SUMMARY OF CAPITAL COSTS FOR EXPANDING RADIOTHERAPY DEPARTMENTS

Savings £M	Expenditure £M	Nett Extra Costs £M
7M	6M - new bunkers 9M - major schemes 3M - minor schemes	
£7M	£18M	£11M

Contrary to our initial expectations, the capital costs of reconfiguring the radiotherapy departments is, therefore, relatively low compared with the routine replacement costs. In fact, over a five year period the normal equipment replacement costs, if all existing small departments were to be maintained, would exceed the costs of creating a smaller number of larger radiotherapy departments. Given that the figure of an additional £11M will also achieve a major quality improvement in the facilities and for patients, particularly at Guy's and the Royal London, we regard this as a modest investment.

Future equipment replacement costs would also be much less, with only 39 megavoltage machines instead of the 63 (megavoltage and deep X-ray machines) currently in service.

Capital charges will also reflect this more economical equipment pattern.

9.6.2 Chemotherapy

A number of the preparation areas are poor, especially at the Middlesex, North Middlesex, Charing Cross and the Royal Marsden (Sutton). Expansion of some treatment areas would also be needed, especially for day cases. Both these are small in volume terms and we calculate that the sum of £3M would be a generous allowance for this work.

9.6.3 Outpatient Areas

Modest refurbishment, rather than structural changes are needed at the Royal Marsden Sutton and the Royal London, and to a lesser extent elsewhere. We propose £2M as an indicative figure.

9.6.4 Wards

We have observed unused wards in every Hospital visited, with the possible exception of the Royal London. We have not allowed therefore for major expenditure for new ward accommodation, except for the relocation costs of specialist haematology facilities. The sum of £4M has been allowed, although the pace of decentralisation of this service could reduce this requirement. (We assume most of the haematology work will continue on its existing sites, even if the radiotherapy units move. There are likely to be one or two exceptions to this, hence the sum indicated).

9.6.5 R & D

This it the most difficult area to cost because the space, equipment and other facilities are not owned or managed by the NHS. However, if the NHS were to fund at least a major element of any relocation costs, a sum of £7M could we believe cover much of what might be required.

9.7 OVERALL CAPITAL COSTS

Overall Costs	£M
Radiotherapy Departments	11
Chemotherapy areas	3
Outpatients	2
Wards, including haematology	4
R & D	7
TOTAL	27

9.8 PROFESSIONAL ISSUES AFFECTED BY CHANGE

It is not an entirely simple matter in professional or care terms to effect substantial changes in referral patterns. Clinics which have operated well to give a good service for years will have built up productive professional liaison and understanding which add to the benefit of the patients. Changes to these need to be carefully thought through at a much more detailed level than we could undertake. The planning of such changes, especially if they are to take place quite quickly, is therefore all important if standards of care are not to suffer. Nevertheless, we believe the changes in outreach clinics tied to particular centres are necessary to improve service co-ordination as well as teaching and research.

SECTION 10.   LIST OF APPENDICES

1.   Terms of Reference.

2.   Membership of the Steering Group and Study Groups.

3.   Profile of 15 London Centres:

      3.1   Staffing
      3.2   Estates
      3.3   Revenue Income

4.   Problems with Cancer Information Systems

5.   Planning Methodolgy Used

6.   New Patients Analysis - Royal Marsden Hospital

7.   Glossary of Terms and Abbreviations

8.   Bibliography

TERMS OF REFERENCE

The Terms of Reference announced by the Minister for Health on 27th February were:-

- To review the literature concerned with the organisation and financing of the specialty.

- To assess the opportunities for prevention and the need for treatment for the diseases usually cared for by the specialty and incorporate views on the likely developments arising from research initiatives, demographic trends, and changes in the incidence or prevalence of disease.

- To define appropriate models of care for the patient at home, in outpatients, in day care facilities, and in hospitals, hospices, and hotels covering all stages of disease, including the management of long term disability.

- To define the criteria for a tertiary centre and specify the service the centre should provide.

- To specify the contribution of individual departments to a multidisciplinary tertiary centre such as neurosciences, and also other departments that should be present on the same site though not part of the centre itself.

- To describe the contribution the tertiary centre would make to teaching undergraduate and postgraduate students and the requirements necessary for a research base.

- To comment on issues of access, quality and timeliness in the provision of care and communication with the patient and relatives, particularly regarding the burden of care that the family will carry.

- To consider the arrangements necessary for collaborating with the social services and voluntary agencies.

- To analyse services currently available in London: the volume and quality of work, and its geographical distribution.

- To bring together these considerations and such other information or advice as is deemed appropriate into a set of proposals for the delivery of care in London.

MEMBERSHIP OF THE STEERING GROUPS AND STUDY GROUPS

STEERING GROUP:

Dr. C.H. Paine, President, Royal College of Radiologists (Chairman)
Mr. M. Bellamy, Chief Executive, Ealing, Hammersmith & Hounslow Health Agency (Co-ordinator)
Professor M. Baker, Regional Director of Research and Development, Yorkshire Regional Health Authority
Professor S.B. Kaye, Professor of Oncology, Glasgow
Professor R. Mansel, Professor of Surgery, Cardiff
Dr. E. Murray, General Practitioner, London
Mrs. G. Oliver, Regional Nurse, Mersey Regional Health Authority
Dr. H. Sanderson, Director, National Casemix Office
Dr. P. Simpson, London Implementation Group
Dr. G. Thorpe, Consultant Physician in Palliative Care, Southampton
Ms. L. Tinckham, Cancer Relief Macmillan Fund

Ms. S. Harris   (Administrator)
Mrs J.M. Embra   (Secretary)

MANPOWER, PLANNING AND EDUCATION AND TRAINING STUDY GROUP:

Ms. P. Oakley (Chairman)
Ms. L. Mullins
Ms. C. Sturdy

EPIDEMIOLOGY STUDY GROUP:

Dr. H. Sanderson (Chairman)
Dr. S. Boyle
Dr. M. Coleman
Mrs. C. Garrett
Dr. L. Laird
Dr. A. Pollock
Dr. J. Raftery

RESEARCH & DEVELOPMENT REVIEW:

Professor M. Baker (Chairman)

PATIENT INFORMATION AND SUPPORT SERVICES
(including Palliative Care) STUDY GROUP:

Ms. L. Tinckham (Chairman)
Mrs K. Turner/Ms S. Harris (Co-ordinators)
Ms. C. Dickens
Ms. J. Gaffin
Ms. A. Hayes
Mrs. J. Millington
Ms. R. Miles
Mrs. G. Oliver
Dr. G. Thorpe
Mr. A. Westall

PRIMARY CARE STUDY GROUP:

Dr. E. Murray (Chairman)
Ms. S. Harris (Co-ordinator)
Dr. J. Austoker
Mrs. M. Brennan
Ms. G. Dunn
Ms. J. McGillivray
Ms. J. Pharoah
Dr. S. Singh
Ms. C. Waugh

TECHNICAL ADVICE AND INFORMATION ANALYSIS STUDY GROUP:

Mr. P. Dick
Mr. J. Dobby
Mr. S. Kirby
Mr. R. Lukacs
Dr. H. Sanderson
Mrs. C. Garrett

FACT FINDING GROUP:

Mr. P. Tankard	-	Estates
Mr. J. Mills		
Mr. D. Blair		
Mr. J. Dobby	-	Manpower
Miss P. Blackbourn	-	Radiotherapy Workload and Facilities
Mr. P. Whiffen	-	Chemotherapy Workload and Facilities
Ms. N. Stoner		

ADVISORS TO THE MANPOWER AND EDUCATION SUB-GROUP

Manpower Data

John Dobby	Non-medical Epidemiologist Ealing, Hounslow and Hammersmith Commissioning Agency

Medical Staff

Professor Charles Easmon	Postgraduate Dean, BPMF
Dr Angela Jones	Associate Director of Public Health, NWTRHA
Dr Alistair Scotland	Director of Public Health, NETHRHA

Nurses

Rachel Hornsby	Oncology Nurse Tutor, Southampton University
Jean Flanagan	Course Leader, Continuing Care, Leeds University
Celia Manson	Advisor in Nursing Practice, RCN
Pam McLinton	Team Leader, Swindon Park Clinic, Luton
Lucy Stewart	Regional Coordinator for Continuing Care, NWTRHA

Therapeutic Radiographers

Peter Smith	Director for Professional and Educational Services, College of Radiographers
Anne Shaw	Principal, West Midlands School of Therapeutic Radiography, Stoke on Trent
Barbara Shaw-Evans	Cancer Services Manager, Bristol General Hospital
Janet High	Principal Lecturer, Division of Clinical Sciences (Radiography), University of Hertfordshire
Diana Whait	Superintendent Radiographer, Mount Vernon Hospital

Medical Physicists

Dr Philip Dendy	President of Institute for Physical Sciences in Medicine
Dr Edwin Aird	Medical Physics Department, Mount Vernon Hospital

Dietitians

Anne Bibbington	Department of Nutrition and Dietetics, Walsgrave Hospital
Maggie Robbinson	British Dietetics Association

Occupational Therapists

Georgina Smith	Education Advisor, College of Occupational Therapists
Beryl Steeden	Head of Professional Affairs, College of Occupational Therapists
Beverley Landreth	Senior Occupational Therapist, Teeside Hospice Care Foundation, Middlesborough

Physiotherapists

Karen Romain	Professional Affairs Officer, Chartered Society of Physiotherapists
Ann Clark	District Physiotherapist, Bedford Hospital NHS Trust

Clinical Psychologists

Lesley Parkinson	District Psychologist, Riverside Health Authority

Pharmacists

Stephen Garner	Chief Pharmacist, University Hospital Trust, Nottingham (Pharmacy Advisor, Nottingham Health Authority)
Phillip Wiffen	Director of Pharmacy Services, Churchill Hospital, Oxford

CURRENT STAFFING AT LONDON CANCER CENTRES (W.T.E.)

| | CONSULTANTS | | | MEDICAL TRAINING POSTS(2) | RADIOGRAPHERS | PHYSICS (ENGINEERS) | NURSES(3) |
	CL.ONC.	MED.ONC.	OTHERS(1)				
North Middx.	2.7	0	1.3	0	12.0	3.8 (1.5)	22.0
UCH/Middlesex	3.1	1.8	3.8	14.0	36.0	8.5 (2.5)	108.4
Royal Free	1.7	1.4	0.4	3.0	13.1	5.0 (3.0)	59.6
St. Mary's	1.5	0	0	0	2.0	0.5 (0)	2.0
Hammersmith	4.7	1.2	N/K	5.5	16.0	4.0 (3.0)	29.72
Charing Cross	5.1	4.4	1.0	11.0	21.5	6.2 (5.0)	57.5
Marsden (Fulham)	2.8	2.0	2.8	10.0	25.6	7.5 (5.0)	198.85
Marsden (Sutton)	5.3	4.0	5.7	23.0	31.0	8.0 (7.0)	136.36
St.Bartholomew's	2.7	3.0	2.7	7.5	18.6	4.5 (2.0)	81.5
Royal London	3.0	2.0	3.6	9.4	18.6	5.25 (4.0)	31.0
Oldchurch	2.7	0	1.1	0	14.1	5.0 (2.0)	6.0
King's							
Guy's	7.7	3.0	N/K	4.0	35.4	7.5 (5.0)	12.0
Thomas'							
Mount Vernon	8.0	0.5	0.3	6.0	25.4	5.7 (6.0)	53.8
London Total	51.0	23.3	22.7	93.4	269.3	71.45 (46.0)	798.73

Notes: (1)   Haemato-Oncology, palliative care and paediatric oncology, excludes surgery posts.
(2)   Senior Registrar and Registrar posts, excluding surgery and haemato-oncology.
(3)   Employed in inpatient, outpatient and day care units, excluding haematology unit staff and surgical ward staff at the Royal Marsden Hospitals.
*   Figure not available

Estate Issues — Review of Cancer Service — Existing Situation

Estate Issues	Unit	UCH/Middx	Royal Free	N.Middx	Kings	Thomas'	Thomas'/Guys	Charing X	R.Marsden	R.Marsden/R.M.Sutton	Barts	Oldchurch	Hammersmith	MVH	St.Marys	R.London	TOTALS
RADIOTHERAPY MACHINES																	
– Linacs	No	3*	2*	1	1	2	1	4*	4*	5	4*	2*	3*	5*	0	3**	40*10 {70 low voltage / 12 high voltage}
– Cobalt	No	2**	1*	2**	1*	1*	1*	1*	1*	1*	0	1*	1*	0	0	1*	14*14
– DXR	No	1*	1*	1*	0	0	1*	1*	0	1*	1*	1	0	0	1*	1*	9*9
– SXR	No	1*	1*	1	0	1*	1*	1*	1*	0		1*	1*	1	1*	2*	13*9
– Afterloading	No	1*	1	1*	1*	1	1	1	2	TBI	0	1	2	1	0	3*	16*5
– Simulators	No	2	1	1	0	2*	0	1	2*	1	1	1	1	2	0	1	16*2
– Planning Systems	No	2	1	1	0	1	1	1	1	2	1	2	1	3	0	2	19
– Existing Value (NBV)	£	0.52m	0.90m	2.34m	N/A	N/A	N/A	5.0m	8.20m	7.98m	N/A	N/A	6.0m	2.5m	MIN	0.85m	15
– Replacement Costs (Each "*" indicates a machine to be replaced by 1998)	£	1.82m	1.20m	1.22m	0.62m	1.07m	0.60m	1.20m	1.45m	0.60m	0.62m	1.10m	1.10m	0.5m	0.20m	1.82m	12m (+installation + VAT)
DIAGNOSTIC EQUIPMENT																	
– MRI/MRS	No	2	1	0	1	0	1	1 (due)	0	1 (COMBINED)	1	0	3	2	1	1	16
– CT	No	2	1	1	1	0	1 (+1/2PET)	2	1	1	2	2	2 (+2PET)	2 (1 CT SIM)	2	2	25
QUALITY OF ACCOMMODATION																	
– R.T.treatment areas		B	B	B	C	B	D	A	B	A	C	D	B	A	D	C	
– Chemotherapy treatment areas		B	A	B	D	B	A	B	A	B	A	C	A	A	D	A	
– OPD waiting areas (dedicated to cancer)		A	B	B	C	B	A (under const)	A	B	B	B	C	A (under const)	A	C/D	B	
– Ward areas	No of beds	B (64)	B (24)	B (30)	B/C (10)	B (49)	B (53)	B (78)	A/B (181)	A/B (184)	B (75)	C (24)	A (24+14)	B (71)	C (12)	B (31)	
– Research labs		A	B	–	C	B	B	A	A	–	B	off site hospice	A	A (Gray L)	–	B	
– Hostel beds	No	14	42	0	0	0	0	1+40 CW	0	6	0	0	0	10 (CHART)	0	16	
RELATIONSHIP TO R.T.TREATMENT																	
– Diagnostic Department		A	A	B	B+	A	A	A	A	A	C	A	B	A	D	C	
– Wards		C	B	B	B	B+	B+	B+	A	B+	C	A	A	A	D	A	
– OPD (Oncology)		D	A	A	A	A	B+	A	A	A	B	A	A	A	C	A	
– other DGH specialities		B	A	B	A	A	A	A	D	D	B	A	A	B	B	A	
ACCESSIBILITY																	
– Sign Posting	Good/Ave/Poor	Ave	Good	Poor	Ave	Good	Poor	Good	Good	Good	Poor	Poor	Ave	Good	Poor	Ave	
– Car parking		Poor	Good	Good	Poor	Poor	Poor	Ave	Poor	Good	Ave	Good	Poor	Good	Poor	Poor	
INVESTMENT IN CANCER SERVICES IN LAST 5 YRS		–	£3.8m	£11m (tender)	£3.6m		incl below	£3m	£45m		£4.3m		£5m	£5.4m	£0.015m	£6m/yr	
WHOLE SITE INVESTMENT		–	£15m		£40m		£190m	£10.8m	£45m		£50m		£64.5m	£15m			

Note: N/A means not available

Note: 1 (being decomm'd July 1993)

1991/92 REVENUE INCOME IN £,000 (EXCLUDING CAPITAL CHARGES) FOR CANCER SERVICES

	Radiotherapy	Chemotherapy	Haematology	Total
UCH/Middlesex	6,299	1,185	5,465	12,949
Royal Free	2,140	764	6,370	9,274
Guy's/Thomas'	4,137	4,922	2,036	11,095
St. Bartholomew's	873	1,226	2,267	4,366
Royal London	1,352	762	2,962	5,076
Charing Cross	3,670	2,254	3,117	9,041
Hammersmith	1,377	3,069	3,681	8,127
Royal Marsden***	14,132*	10,412*	17,837*	42,381
King's	1,085*	799*	1,369*	3,253
Oldchurch	1,085*	800*	957	2,842
Mount Vernon	2,503*	1,845*	3,160*	7,508**
North Middlesex	809	1,038	176	2,023
	39,462	29,076	49,397	117,935

Source - Information provided by Units

*   Split estimated using the average from those Centres that showed separate figures.

**   1992/93 figures

***   Both Branches

Commentary

The split of income between the three service areas (Radiotherapy, Chemotherapy and Haematology) was not provided by all units; for this and other reasons we therefore believe it needs to be treated with caution.

The overall total for each unit, we regard as a more useful indicator, but we have again treated it with caution, and only taken it to build up an estimate of the total spend on specialist cancer services for the 15 centres.

PROBLEMS WITH CURRENT INFORMATION SYSTEMS

Significant difficulties were encountered by the Cancer Services Review Group in securing adequate and reliable data on which to base factual comparisons of Cancer Centres, and projections of demand for services and future workload. This difficulty is consistent with that found by other groups carrying out large scale cancer studies, e.g. the 1990 Review of Cancer Services in Scotland.

The difficulties encountered can be broadly summarised as follows:-

Workload Data

Some Centres generate case notes for all patients seen in DGHs i.e. DGH wards and outpatients, with all such patients being counted within the total of new referrals to that Centre per annum. Other Centres rely on the host DGH to generate the case notes for such outpatient referrals, only initiating their own case notes once the patient is seen at the specialist Centre itself.

The definition of a new patient varies between Centres. In some a patient attending for a subsequent course of radiotherapy treatment (if this is given more than 8 weeks after the first course), is counted as a new patient. In others the patient will be recorded as a follow-up if the treatment is given within the same year. In yet others, a patient is only counted as 'new' if he or she presents later in life with a second (new) cancer, but not if there is even years later a recurrence of the first cancer.

Regular ward attendees are frequently recorded in in-patient bed days, distorting some Centres' bed utilisation figures.

Patients admitted under a surgeon who subsequently, but during the same in-patient episode, undergo specialist cancer treatment, are usually recorded as a Surgical Finished Consultant Episode, with the oncologist specialist input not being separately recorded, except by the Cancer Centre especially if radiotherapy is given.

There is little reliable data available on case mix within cancer services, although some centre do maintain their own disease index, regarding this as the only way to monitor their activity and clinical practice.

There is little or no data available on patient flows for radiotherapy, which is mainly performed on an outpatient basis. The majority of flow data available relates to in-patient bed utilisation, and a confused picture exists between surgical and medical (oncology) bed use for cancer patients.

Cancer Registry Data

The Thames Cancer Registry estimates that approximately 10% of all cancers are not registered.

Most of these patients are thought to be treated at home with rapidly fatal cancers for which hospital care is inappropriate. A few will have slipped through the registration system in hospitals and will have had their cancers cured. The figure excludes non-melanoma skin cancers.

A further 17% are registered only from death certificates, these patients most usually being those who die within 2-3 years of their treatment.

Whilst, therefore Cancer Registry data have been valuable to the Review, it is strongly recommended that recording systems be improved especially at the interface between clinicians and the outposted cancer registry staff who work in hospitals. The larger cancer centres we propose should in future have the facilities to record and download these data directly to the cancer registry, so saving cost and improving accuracy and timeliness.

Financial Data

There is no common methodology applied to the calculation of specialty costs and wide variations are found in unit costs and prices for cancer treatment and care. We strongly recommend that work currently in progress between the National Casemix Office and others on Health Related Groups and their costings, be taken forward to develop such a methodology which can be owned by clinicians, service directors and managers jointly, and used in the contracting process of the future.

PLANNING METHODOLOGY USED

ESTIMATING THE FUTURE NEED/DEMAND FOR CANCER SERVICES

Our overall estimate is that the number of patients requiring cancer treatment will increase by 15% during the next decade, predominantly due to the increasing number of elderly people in the population, but also due to increased incidence of some cancers. This is broadly in line with projections made in other recent reviews of cancer carried out elsewhere in the U.K.

The Thames Cancer Registry have analysed data for South West Thames for 1975 to 1989 and have estimated an increase in the incidence of cancer of 10% over the next decade. The Review Group also gathered information from other Centres in the U.K. and this indicated that between 1989 and 1992 there were wide variations in the rate of increase in new radiotherapy attendances.

The Review Group felt that, in the light of the significant reorganisation of services required to effect the optimum pattern of cancer services, it was more appropriate to plan for service provision in 1996/7 based on the higher of the above projections.

ESTIMATING THE NEED FOR RADIOTHERAPY EQUIPMENT

The estimates used in a number of recent studies elsewhere in the U.K. have been reviewed. The existing utilisation of equipment in London Units has also been examined. We have then taken the projected increase in incidence, the population to be served and assumed an improved level of machine utilization, to one approaching that already achieved elsewhere.

However, given the presence, taking the 15 London Centres, of a volume of equipment substantially in excess of the projected need based on studies elsewhere in the U.K. as well as our own analysis, we have assumed that little new equipment will need to be purchased in the next five years with some machines being relocated. This will still leave the proposed London Centres with a significantly higher level of major treatment machines than elsewhere in the country. This will allow for the impact of:-

- Some unmet need being in future referred for treatment.

- Some case-mix variations.

- The working of new machines being slower due to more complex in safety terms and allowing asymetrical treatment areas.

- The possible additional impact of new treatment regimes like Chart.

1991 - 1992 NEW PATIENTS ENTERED INTO THERAPEUTIC CLINICAL TRIALS BY UNIT

	Total New Cases	Malignant Diagnosis	Available For Research	Approved Research Protocol	Referred Elsewhere	Overseas
BREAST	3697	1352	1049	710 (68%)	147	156
CHEMOPREVENTION *	1098	0	1098	147 (13%)	0	0
GYNAECOLOGY	558	493	368	230 (63%)	61	64
HEAD AND NECK	679	344	238	84 (35%)	39	67
PALL/PSYCHO MEDICINE **	549	549	549	188 (35%)	7	6
SARCOMA	212	174	124	51 (41%)	24	26
SKIN & MELANOMA	782	434	338	142 (42%)	64	32
UROLOGY & TESTIS	737	554	437	192 (44%)	54	63
CLIN PHARMACOLOGY	71	71	67	41 (61%)	4	0
GI TRACT	717	675	464	311 (67%)	155	56
LEUKAEMIA	196	135	75	70 (93%)	12	48
LYMPHOMA	306	269	159	88 (55%)	30	80
LUNG	618	598	390	173 (44%)	135	73
MYELOMA	72	67	43	30 (70%)	12	12
NEURO-ONCOLOGY	231	195	136	80 (59%)	27	32
PAEDIATRICS ***	224	106	63	62 (98%)	17	26
THYROID ****	157	66	46	16 (35%)	5	15

* Women thought to be at higher than normal risk of developing breast cancer only a few are eligible for the chemoprevention study with Tamoxifen.
** All these patients are internally referred.
*** Many children with or without malignancy are referred for special investigation only.
**** Non malignant cases are referred for ^{131}I therapy.

GLOSSARY OF TERMS AND ABBREVIATIONS

Clinical oncology The use and practice of radiotherapy and oncology in treating cancer. Clinical oncologists were previously known as radiotherapists and oncologists.

Medical oncology The use and development of chemotherapy, biological modalities and gene therapy in treating cancer; either as single agents or in conjunction with other modalities.

Surgery Includes diagnostic surgery (the removal of tissue for diagnosis and staging of the illness) and the removal of tumours. Depending on the nature of the cancer, surgery may be performed by general surgeons in local acute hospitals who have developed an interest in cancer, or by surgeons who specialise partly or entirely in oncology.

Haemato-oncology The diagnosis and treatment of blood related malignancy and some associated solid tumours.

Allogeneic Bone marrow transplants From a sibling.

Autologous Bone marrow replacement using the patient's own, stored, marrow.

Palliative Medicine Comprehensive care and support for patients with progressive, advanced, incurable disease, and for their families. Its goal is the achievement of the best possible quality of life.

Beds Different levels of nursing care are required in cancer centres;- intensive care (eg. for BMT), acute wards, 5 day wards, hostel accommodation (i.e. support at hand), hotel accommodation (warden supervision only).

Family Used in its widest sense to represent all people who are significant in a patient's life. May include partners, blood relations, children, friends, neighbours and other carers.

Inner/Outer London As defined in Sir Bernard Tomlinson's review of London health services. (We have taken Outer London as being within the M25 but excluding central London)

ABBREVIATIONS

BMT	-	Bone Marrow Transplantation
CCE	-	Completed Consultant Episode
CHART	-	Continuous Hyperfractionated and Accelerated Radiotherapy
CHC	-	Community Health Council
CHSC	-	Chelsea Health Sciences Centre
CRC	-	Cancer Research Campaign
CRMF	-	Cancer Relief Macmillan Fund
CT	-	Computerised Tomography
DGH	-	District General Hospital (or local acute hospital)
DHA	-	District Health Authority (or local health purchasing agency)
DoH	-	Department of Health
FHSA	-	Family Health Services Authority
HEA	-	Health Education Authority
HOTN	-	"Health of the Nation" White Paper (1992)
ICR	-	Institute of Cancer Research
ICRF	-	Imperial Cancer Relief Fund
ITU	-	Intensive Therapy Unit
Linac	-	Linear Accelerator
MRC	-	Medical Research Council
MRI	-	Magnetic Resonance Imaging
NHSME	-	NHS Management Executive
OPCS	-	Office of Population, Censuses and Surveys
PET	-	Positron Emission Tomography
R & D	-	Research and Development
RPMS	-	Royal Postgraduate Medical School (Hammersmith)
RT	-	Radiotherapy
SELRC	-	South East London Radiotherapy Centre
SHA	-	Special Health Authority
SHO	-	Senior House Officer
UFC	-	University Funding Council
UICC	-	Union International Contre Le Cancer

BIBLIOGRAPHY

The Steering Group consulted a wide range of reviews and papers relating to cancer services. The group also considered the many responses from Royal Colleges and their Faculties to Sir Bernard Tomlinson's Review of London Health Services. The documents are too numerous to list in full but it was thought that an abbreviated bibliography might be of interest and use.

Chamberlain, J
"The Feasibility of Indicators and Targets for Cancer Control." (Oct. 1991)

Department of Health
"The Health of the Nation - Key Area Handbook: Cancers." (Jan. 1993)

Dische, S.
"London's Cancer Services: A consideration of the present and future need for the care of patients with cancer in London and South East England." (Jan.1993)

Doll, R.
"Are We Winning the War Against Cancer? A Review in Memory of Keith Durrant." (Clinical Oncology, 1992, 4:257-266)

Health Services Manpower Review
"The Care of the Dying." (Papers presented at a National Conference held in London, Jan.1987)

The Hospice Information Service, St.Christopher's Hospice
"Provision of Hospice Services in the Thames Regions." (Jan.1993)

The International Commission on Radiation Protection
"Protection of the Patient in Radiation Therapy." (May 1984)

NW Thames Regional Health Authority
"Review of the Cancer Treatment Services in the North West Thames Region." (May 1987)

Northern Regional Health Authority
"Cancer Services in the Northern Region; A Report to the Regional Medical Committee." (Sept.1992)

Rees, G.J.G., Deutsch, G.P., Dunlop, P.R.C. and Priestman, T.J.
"Clinical Oncology Services to District General Hospitals: Report of a Working Party of the Royal College of Radiologists" (Clinical Oncology, 1991 3:41-45)

The Royal College of Physicians and the Royal College of Radiologists Joint Council for Clinical Oncology
"Reducing Delays in Cancer Treatment: Improving Quality Control, Some Treatment Targets." (Jan.1993)

The Royal College of Radiologists
"Cancer Care and Treatment Services: Advice for Purchasers and Providers." (Sept.1991)

The Royal College of Radiologists
"Making the best use of a Department of Clinical Radiology: Guidelines for Doctors" (1993)

The Scottish Office
"Management of Non-Surgical Cancer Services in Scotland." (Feb.1992)

Sikora, K. & Waxman, J.
"Going for Cure: A strategy for London's cancer services in the next century." (April 1992)

Sikora, K. & Waxman, J.
"Cancer Services for London: A Way Forward." (Jan.1993)

South Western Regional Health Authority
"Cancer Services in the South Western Region." (March 1990)

Standing Medical Advisory Committee
"Acute Services for Cancer." (July 1984)

Standing Medical Advisory Committee and Standing Nursing & Midwifery Advisory Committee Joint Report
"The Principles and Provision of Palliative Care." (1992)

Strickland, P.
"Patient Norms for Linear Accelerators." (May 1981)

Thames Cancer Registry
Cancer in the Thames Regions 1987-89 (Dec.1992)

UICC "Guidelines for Developing a Comprehensive Cancer Centre." (Geneva 1980)

Ware, J.E.
"Measuring patients' views: the optimum outcome measure" (British Medical Journal, 306, page 1429 - 30, 29th May 1993)

Welsh Health Planning Forum
"Protocol for Investment in Health Gain: Cancers." (Dec.1990)

Wilkie, T.
"Perilous Knowledge: The Human Genome Project and its implications" (Faber & Faber Ltd., London 1993)

Williams, C.J.
"Introducing new treatments for cancer: practical, ethical and legal problems." (John Wiley & Sons, Chichester 1992)

Printed in the United Kingdom for HMSO.
Dd.296539, 6/93, C35, 3396/4, 5673, 249611.